LIFE, NUTRITION, AND WELLNESS 101

LIFE, NUTRITION, AND WELLNESS 101

A Holistic Approach with a Philosophical Twist

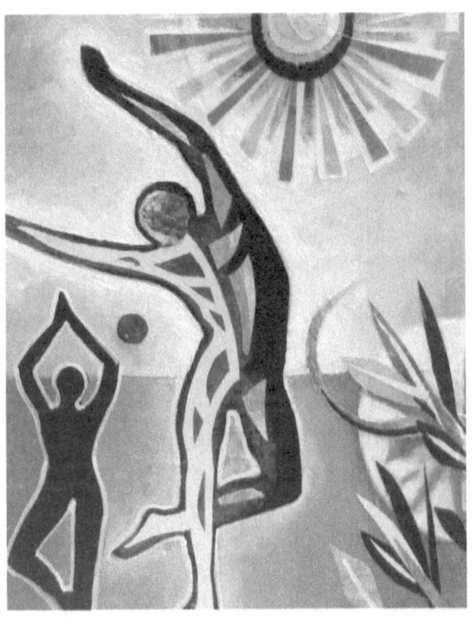

TONY PATRICK NOREIGA, DPM

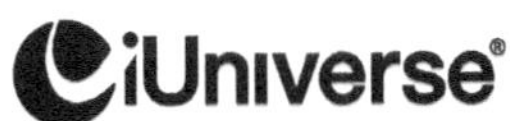

LIFE, NUTRITION, AND WELLNESS 101
A HOLISTIC APPROACH WITH A PHILOSOPHICAL TWIST

iUniverse books may be ordered through booksellers or by contacting:

iUniverse
1663 Liberty Drive
Bloomington, IN 47403
www.iuniverse.com
844-349-9409

Because of the dynamic nature of the internet, any web addresses or links contained in this book may have changed since publication and may no longer be valid. The views expressed in this work are solely those of the author and do not necessarily reflect the views of the publisher, and the publisher hereby disclaims any responsibility for them.

Any people depicted in stock imagery provided by Getty Images are models, and such images are being used for illustrative purposes only.
Certain stock imagery © Getty Images.

ISBN: 978-1-6632-1536-9 (sc)
ISBN: 978-1-6632-1535-2 (hc)
ISBN: 978-1-6632-1537-6 (e)

Library of Congress Control Number: 2021900478

Print information available on the last page.

iUniverse rev. date: 02/11/2021

To the notable Sadhguru, a renowned teacher, author, visionary, mystic, spiritualist, and yogi.

Health is wealth.

—Ralph Waldo Emerson, 1860
(said with simplicity and elegance)

CONTENTS

PREFACE

Life, Nutrition, and Wellness 101 is my second published work. As I delve into this subject of interest, I am without the authoritative credentials or special accolades in the field of nutrition. My background is in podiatric medicine and surgery. However, I do like to consider myself an enthusiast and a devoted student of life, health, and wellness. I am always delighted to share.

Together with my clinical background, I have come to realize how fortunate I am to have spent my formative years living on the Caribbean island of Trinidad and Tobago.

What would be classified as third world poverty on one hand, in the long run was a blessing in disguise. This unembellished lifestyle (usually barely clothed) also endowed me with a spirited sense of appreciation for life as it currently is. In addition, I was bestowed with a hands-on familiarity with many of the fruits, herbs, and vegetables introduced within the text.

As a health connoisseur, I have relied on my experiences, along with a stockpile of personal notes on life, nutrition, and wellness, to bring this succinct book to fruition.

The beauty of differing voices is that ideas, thoughts, stories, or data are rarely valued and adopted by way of a single voice. As we each perceive information in a distinct fashion, it is my hope that this platform will provide some level of light for the unsettled population niche.

ACKNOWLEDGMENTS

You'll note that I have humbly dedicated this book to Sadhguru. He has sublimely inspired me, through his workshops and presentations, to complete this publication. My gratitude to him is beyond measure.

Special thanks goes to my three sons:

- To Sterling, a soccer and hip-hop aficionado, who seems to gracefully challenge me equal to himself.
- To Isaiah, an attentive listener and humble onward achiever.
- To Lil Tony, grounded in faith and a fist full of love.
- Special shout-out to my illustrator, an international artist, Glenn Roopchand. My philosophical mentor and family inspiration.

And special thanks to my darling wife of thirty-seven years, Rebecca, for her unconditional support for us all.

INTRODUCTION

This manuscript is designed to shed some light on the fact that "good health" is beyond appearance and equally essential to the mental, physical, and spiritual properties of the body. Our bodies function in harmony (or disharmony) with each organ system, which in turn interrelates with our environment. This understanding can be indistinguishable to our daily food consumption. More often than not, food choices are highlighted over exercise, and exercise is perpetuated over a positive mindset. However, at minimum, all three entities should have equal merit when it comes to health and leading a balanced lifestyle.

If I may impress anything upon you, it's that there is no quick and easy fix to full health. Without question, the healthier the body and mind, the richer life is destined to be. Nevertheless, how a person chooses to live or where one chooses to direct his or her energy should be unwaveringly respected. First, focusing on full health may not be one's desire. Second, respect and understanding should be unyielding, as we are not always ready or equipped to modify our lifestyles at any given period.

This book is written as a venture to bridge the gap in some way. *Life, Nutrition, and Wellness* is wholeheartedly given the accompanying modifier *101*. As such, it is likely to appeal to individuals like myself, who have yet to master the basics and can humbly appreciate added inspiration. This information may not be novel, but the timing and manner by which it is expressed will hopefully raise readers' consciousness and encourage wellness.

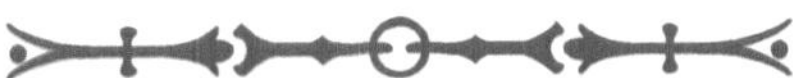

PART I

FUNDAMENTALS

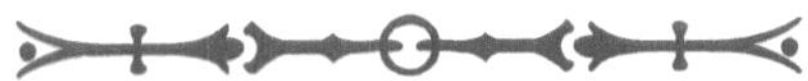

CHAPTER 1

HUMAN OVERVIEW

If you dissolve or disintegrate the human body, the following is what results. Microscopically, there are three fundamental elements—hydrogen, oxygen, and carbon.

There are three thousand trillion, trillion atoms in the average human. This makes fifty trillion cells. All of us are unique due to the twenty-three pairs of distinct chromosomes in our cells. Each pair of chromosomes contains DNA (genes), which gives humans the various characteristics (traits) we possess.

From a more sizeable perspective, there are about seventy-eight body organs, which are specifically grouped to form eleven systems. The systems unite to form one organism, which is the human body.

Of the seventy-eight organs in the human body, there are some with which we all are familiar:

- skin
- kidneys
- heart
- arteries
- muscles
- liver
- tongue
- gallbladder

- skeleton
- pancreas
- veins
- brain
- intestine
- larynx
- eyes
- urinary bladder
- stomach
- lungs
- bone marrow
- lymph nodes

CHAPTER 2

GMO

When it comes to GMOs, there are three important questions: What are they? How do they impact us? And how should we respond?

Genetically Modified Organisms (GMOs) are currently an inevitable part of our food choices. With economics as a key impetus, along with our population explosion, food demands, and technological advancements, GMOs are here to stay.

A handful of major companies essentially control the chemical pesticides and GMOs that have become part of the world's food chain. While farmers' primary objective is to attain high crop yields, their greatest hurdle has been the destruction of crops by insects.

Chemical insecticides alone solved only half the problem, as the vegetation also suffered from utilization of these chemical insecticides.

This gave rise to the technology of biological engineering, which involves modifying the crop seeds to withstand high quantities of pesticides. This so-called solution has created our current market of genetically modified organisms—GMO foods.

How is this done? Basically, certain plant genes are extracted, spliced, added, or interchanged so that the planted vegetation is resistant to an abundance of pesticides, without harm to the plants. While this advancement has accommodated large crop yields, we pay a price in the form of adverse effects of chemically-induced food items. Drawbacks to GMO usage are not limited to new strains of insects and toxicity to the human body. Whether the repercussions are subtle or obvious, allergies or cancer, GMO consumption impacts us in good (high crop yield) and not so good ways (as noted).

The most common GMO-induced foods and vegetation are corn, alfalfa (for grass-fed animals), sugar, tomatoes, papayas, whitish sugar beets, and many others. These food commodities account for high crop yields. High crop yields translate to high cash crops. In addition, GMO products are commonly used in animal farms, at fast food restaurants, and in essentially all processed foods.

So where do we go from here? This introductory information is designed for personal empowerment. We can raise our level of awareness and understanding and, thereby, make sensible food choices as best as we are able.

Limiting the details and without diverting from my core purpose, one can envision that the implications of GMO are not limited to high quantities of insecticides used in fruits and vegetables. GMO hybrid foods caters for seedless fruits, enlarged produce, nonseasonal availability, increase sugar content along with a lowering of nutritional value and other adverse effects which accompany such GMO modifications. Scientific, business, and administrative entities all have an interest, as GMO technology is applicable to disease intervention, transhumanism, and population management.

CHAPTER 3

THE JOURNEY

In deciding what to do and what not to do, we need not stress ourselves over exclusives such as what's "right" or what's "wrong." Such parallels never see unity but, instead, perpetuate separateness and disenlightenment. Instead, we can consider and maneuver ourselves according to what is most beneficial to us all.

Good nutrition brings you well-being, just as it does for everyone around you. Health and wellness can be thought of as a collective effort involving the mind and the body. This includes what you consume, what you think, your vibes, and your life choices.

Most of us take good measures to stay healthy, yet we find ourselves confronted with unwarranted ailments. We may ask ourselves, Why me? Many factors can contribute to the ailments that conflict us. Among these are environment, lifestyle, personal choices, stress, mental solidity, and genetic predisposition. However, even with genetic predisposition, in most adult cases, environment or lifestyle habits play a key role. Predisposition, more often than not, needs a specific risk factor for that condition to materialize. Once again, the vast majority of adult cancer cases have no hereditary association. That said, it essentially behooves us to pay increased attention to what we have control of.

If we're unable or simply decline to take control, we can look within or strive to have a positive outlook.

Approximately 90 percent of all (noninfectious) diseases can be avoided through sustained holistic health, plant-based nutrition, and wellness of our minds and bodies.

Health and fitness is a journey to participate in and appreciate throughout our life's process. It is not a task, a job, or an absolute. It's an activity of transformation or lifestyle that is real. It is a movement by which the body and mind becomes in sync with self and nature.

During this journey of holistic health and nutrition, our body cells become renewed through "new growth" and development. This cellular and organ alteration may take a year or five years, as it is dependent on effort, mindset, genetics, and the energy of the individual.

CHAPTER 4

SUPERFOODS

Briefly speaking, it is my belief that superfoods are essentially all plant-based, natural consumable foods. Yes, some foods do have greater quantities of nutrients. However, most food groups are super in terms of our need for them and when consumed in a palatable and suitable fashion. This is where inclusiveness and food varieties are compelling.

For all intents and purposes, superfoods are food choices that are rich in nutrients and highly beneficial to the human body.

One may classify superfoods by considering the dozens of foods that are strong in antioxidants and provide numerous health benefits.

Alternatively, one could simply say that organic vegetables, herbs, spices, and fruits are all superfoods.

CHAPTER 5

ANTIOXIDANTS AND FREE RADICALS

Information that seemed complexed or far-fetched yesterday is commonplace or obvious today.

Antioxidants and *free radicals* are words we may or may not be familiar with. What are they? And where do they come from? Free radicals are the bad guys. They are chemical compounds that are derived from the environment or from the foods we eat. They are most abundant in red meat, alcohol, cigarettes, fast foods, sugars, fat and oils, and the environment.

Free radicals can destroy or damage our body cells. Stress also triggers (through the release of hormones) the detachment of free radicals.

Antioxidants are the good guys. They are food nutrients (chemical compounds) that eradicate or neutralize free radicals. Most vegetables, herbs, fruits, and many spices are loaded with antioxidants. They include cinnamon, citrus, honey, carrots, kale, sweet potatoes, watercress, avocados, broccoli, pineapple, and ginger, just to name a few.

In essence, antioxidants are from nutrient-rich, plant-based foods, while free radicals are from other foods.

CHAPTER 6

BEYOND OPTIMISM

All life forms have energy.
Our body cells have energy.
Our body cells reverberate.
Reverberations produce sounds.
Our thoughts are a form of reverberations.
Our reverberations resonate, as our thoughts resonate.
Our positive and negative thoughts resonate, sound off, and return similar vibrations.
Beware and be aware—we are how we think.

PART II
FOOD VARIETIES

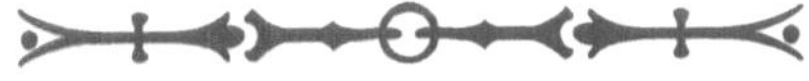

CHAPTER 7

ADAM'S ALE
THE WATER WE DRINK

Water is the most precious consumable food resource on earth.

- Water regulates the earth's temperature.
- About 70 percent of planet Earth is occupied by water.
- About 70 percent of all fresh water is trapped in glaciers (30 percent is underground).
- About 70 percent of our brains (and 60 percent of our bodies) is water.
- About 70 percent of all the world's available fresh water is utilized for farming.

Water (H_2O as a balanced unit) is also known as the blood of life, virgin juice, universal solvent, or Adam's ale. However, water's elemental forms (hydrogen and oxygen) are quite toxic to the body. Water can dissolve more substances than any other liquid.

This precious resource is matched only by its twin sister, alkaline water. One of the many benefits of water is to neutralize acids in the human body. Science has devised a scale to determine if a substance is neutral, acidic, or alkaline. This scale is known as the pH scale and ranges from zero to fourteen.

Water is considered neutral and is valued at 7. If a substance has a pH value between 0 and 6, it is considered acidic, and substances valued between 8 and 14 are alkaline (basic). In the stomach, acid is extremely essential to aid in the breakdown (digestion or metabolism) of food. However, excess body acids from foods or stress have negative effects. Excess acids are directly linked to inefficient muscle activity, mucus accumulation, inflammation, acid reflux, and various other diseases, including cancer and death.

Some *acidic foods* include dairy, coffee, garlic, alcohol, meats, sugar, processed foods, soft drinks, and fried foods.

Food substances that are neutral or alkaline are vegetables, water, herbs, most noncitrus fruits, and others. Alkaline foods are very well tolerated by the human body.

Incidentally, disease processes are unlikely to thrive in an alkaline state in the human body.

Water, among its other functions, enhances blood circulation, prevents dehydration, dilutes digestive (stomach) juices, cleanses our bodies, and keeps our electrolytes (such as sodium and potassium) ions in balance.

If possible, each and every day, enjoy several glasses of this life-sustaining resource. If this is a bit challenging, flavor it up and alkaline it like this: Each morning, fill a glass container with about five glasses of water. Add seven heads of clove and one lime or lemon cut into pieces.

Let it sit and settle. Purchase a glass-sized copper drinking mug. Enjoy this aromatic, flavored alkaline water during the course of the day. It is good at room temperature.

CHAPTER 8

HERBS AND SPICES

Herbs and spices go hand in hand as plant-based, disease-fighting aromatics. They complement each other, as they are both highly nutrient rewarding. In addition, they are interchangeable as herbal teas or seasonings. There may be no further need to purchase expensive, processed herbal teas. Your home pantry is likely to have it all. Here are a few specific spices:

- cumin (*geera*)
- curry
- saffron
- cilantro
- shadow beni
- coriander

A list of the many interchangeable spices and herbs that are rich in phytochemicals (antioxidants) and serve the dual purpose of seasoning food and making herbal tea includes:

- ginger
- parsley
- sage
- peppermint
- barley

- basil
- turmeric
- dill
- rosemary
- Kaffir lime leaves
- oregano
- cloves
- bay leaves
- hibiscus
- rose hip
- orange peel
- dandelion
- lemon (fever) grass

CHAPTER 9

SOYBEANS

Soybeans are the second most abundant US crop after corn. The United States and Brazil are the two world leaders in soybean production. Almost all soy and corn are genetically modified organisms (GMOs).

Soy and soybean products are available in abundance. They include milk, soybeans, nuts, oil, tofu, miso, tempeh (fermented soy cakes), soy burgers, pills, hot dogs, soy sauce, yogurts, cheese and more. Soy is very nutritious due to its high protein content. Soy is also low in cholesterol (saturated fats).

Soy is classified as nothing short of a superfood due to its richness of high-density nutrients and because it's a plant-based food.

However, soy has also been tarnished by possible links to breast and uterine cancer. This association arose due to the presence of phytoestrogens. Phytoestrogens resemble estrogen hormones. Consequently, they were thought to be linked to estrogen-related diseases.

Nonetheless, further investigation and research have dismissed this notion. Apparently, these phytoestrogens are indigenous to the base plant soy. As such, it responds completely different in the human being. Many sources, including the American Cancer Society and the American Institute of Cancer Research, have outlined that soy is safe and that the health benefits outweigh any potential risk. Let it be known that prior to the 1960s, soy was not used as a food source for human consumption in the United States. Instead, it was primarily utilized for production of industrial products and later for livestock.

CHAPTER 10

PROTEIN BUILDERS

The alphabet is to sentences what amino acids are to protein. Amino acids are the foundation or building block of proteins. There are twenty of them. Nine are manufactured by the body, and eleven come strictly from our diet.

We get most of our protein from plants or meat, although most animals get their protein from plants as well. Plants provide all the raw, natural, less-contaminated, and nutritious protein we ever need. Plants are able to produce these amino acids (proteins) directly from the synthesis of four essential components. These substances are sunlight, soil, water, and nitrogen gas from the air.

Proteins are needed for tissue repair and new cell growth. Although meats generally provide more protein per equal size serving of vegetables, the body works twice as hard to metabolize meat. This accounts for the sluggish, heavy feeling we experience upon completing a meaty meal.

Over the decades, we have been told that meats (steaks and seafood) are a sort of status symbol. This notion actually dates back to the days when hunting was a fundamental way of life. To this day, we are conditioned to believe that meat, fish, poultry, and cheese dishes are the central part of a meal. This is traditionally referred to as "the main course." Consequently, it may be difficult to habituate oneself to a plant-based diet.

Be that as it may, the following list includes high-protein foods for meat eaters (left) and nonmeat eaters (right):

- lean chicken / firm soy tofu
- pork / lentils
- tuna / artichokes
- beef / peas
- low-fat yogurt / soybeans
- eggs / dark green vegetables
- cheeses / sweet corn
- seafood / seeds, fruit, and nuts
- milk / mushrooms

CHAPTER 11

SWEET CRYSTALS

Let's start with a few facts on sugar:

- Sugar can be defined as a sweet molecule ($C_{12}H_{22}O_{11}$) made by plants with the aid of sunlight.
- Sugar, similar to stress, alcohol, salt, fat, toxic chemicals, and microorganisms, is often the prime suspect in diseases.
- Common diseases linked to sugar include diabetes, heart disease, liver disease, tooth disease, and obesity.
- Sugar is a carbohydrate, which is composed of glucose and fructose.
- Sugar is used by every cell in the body, but cancer cells are known to utilize more.
- Approximately 75 percent of all processed foods have added sugar.
- The average American consumes approximately a pound each week.

How does an individual consume so much extra sugar? Sugar is added to the diet both directly by choice and indirectly by consuming processed and fast foods. Manufacturers use a variety of terms to camouflage the sugar contents of food items. Here are some names used in lieu of "sugar":

- agave
- ethyl maltol
- raw sugar
- corn sugar
- coconut sugar
- crystalline sugar
- maltose
- brown rice syrup
- molasses
- cane sugar
- muscovado sugar
- caramel
- diastatic malt
- sucrose
- dextran
- sweetener
- fluoride crystals
- sugar crystals
- fructose
- galactose
- fruit juice
- beet sugar
- icing
- grape sugar
- golden syrup
- confectioner's sugar
- granulated sugar

For most adults, 7 teaspoons (35 grams or 150 calories) of sugar a day is far sufficient for the body.

Here are some natural sweeteners to consider:

- agave
- coconut palms
- maple syrup
- sugarcane liquid
- honey
- stevia
- monk fruit

These natural sugars metabolize more easily and slowly, which creates a more gradual rise in blood sugar levels.

Unlike natural sugars, refined sugars, synthetic sugars, and processed sugars metabolize with more of a rush. In addition, cravings for sweets arise due to a similar physiological (bodily) response observed in sugars as observed in drugs such cocaine.

CHAPTER 12

THANKS TO THE BEES

Bees are a vital force toward the contribution of agricultural pollination. The first documented beehive traces back to the ancient Egyptians thousands of years ago. Honey was used as a currency and also as a medicinal substance. Honey was once one of the world's most valued consumables. Europeans used it in recipes and as their chief source of sweeteners.

Honey is made naturally from the nectar of flowers. The bees collect the sweet nectar, digest it, and then regurgitate it into well-structured honeycombs that comprise beehives. The bees repeatedly fan their wings as the water evaporates. The final product is a thick, sweet residue referred to as honey.

It has been scientifically established that honey has antibacterial properties. It may crystalize, but it's unlikely to spoil. It may also serve as an energy booster and is inherently a good antioxidant.

CHAPTER 13

BITTER FOODS

*B*itter is only one of five essential taste sensations (receptors) on our tongue. The other sensations are sweet, sour, salty, and pungent. Pungent means hot or quite spicy, which is, in actuality, a painful nerve sensation, rather than a taste receptor. Anyway, all five taste receptors or sensations contribute to a wholesome experience.

Bitter foods help to provide a magnitude of health benefits and protection against development of diseases. They help to maximize the absorption of nutrients by means of their plant-based chemicals. These superior antioxidant compounds include catechins, carotenoids, minerals, polyphenols, flavonoids, vitamins, and phytochemicals. This explains why bitter foods are *true superfoods*. They are not popular culinary dishes but are substantiated by medical research to provide anti-inflammatory and anticancer properties. They are also effective in reducing or maintaining a more normalized blood sugar and, furthermore, provide protection against gastrointestinal (stomach) infections.

Dark green vegetables and most herbs are the common foods of this category. Here is a list of some bitter foods to consider:

- artichokes
- saffron
- radishes
- sesame seeds
- arugula
- herbs
- dandelion greens
- kale
- cranberries
- broccoli
- brussel sprouts
- citrus peels
- bitter melon
- cocoa

Note: Although the taste may not be initially tolerable for your pallet, ultimate health benefits are obtained when these bitter foods are consumed in their natural state, steamed, or brewed.

CHAPTER 14

SALT PEARLS

Salt is a highly abundant compound, which is composed of sodium (Na^+) ions and chloride (Cl^-) ions. Salt is a principal component in every cell of the human body. In humans, salt is paramount in regulating body fluids, pivotal in controlling our human senses, and crucial for adequate muscle function. In addition, salt helps to regulate blood pressure. It's instrumental for proper functioning of the kidneys and valuable to other organs.

Equally important, one must be mindful that high or excess salt in the body is often the prime suspect for hypertension.

Like most substances or food sources, salt—either in excess or when there is a deficiency—leads to unwarranted ailments, disease, or death.

Currently and historically, salt is used as a natural food preservative due to its antibacterial and protective characteristics. Salt is harvested by means of two principal origins. These two birthplaces are the evaporation of saltwater and salt mine reservoirs. Although there are several salt designations (table salt, pink salt, kosher salt, Celtic salt and fleur de sol), all are basically the same. The primary distinction is the presence or absence of iodine.

Plain table salt is the most fine or delicate, the most commonly used, and contains iodine. Iodine is an essential nonmetal element our bodies require but cannot naturally produce.

Kosher salt is a coarse or rough salt without the added iodine.

Himalayan salt is a rock salt extracted from the Punjab region of Pakistan. This salt has a pink hue due to its diverse mineral content, along with some impurities.

A last word on iodized salt. Iodine is added to salt to assist the body in manufacturing the thyroid hormone. Iodine is necessary for adults and infants. When Iodine is adequately consumed from other food items, iodized salt becomes less needed. Although most plant foods and meats have some Iodine, there are many foods that are rich in iodine content. Some iodine rich foods are:

- seafood
- seaweeds (kelp)
- kale
- dairy products
- cranberries
- boiled eggs
- navy beans
- lima beans

CHAPTER 15

VITAMINS AND MINERALS

Vitamins are substances needed for proper development and function of our body cells. There are approximately thirteen essential vitamins, each serving specific bodily functions.

Our body breaks down, absorbs, and utilizes the various vitamins for different purposes. Vitamins are absorbed in our bodies by fats or by water. Hence, we have categorized them as fat-soluble vitamins and water-soluble vitamins.

FAT-SOLUBLE VITAMINS

Fat-soluble vitamins (FSVs) require body fat to be dissolved for adequate absorption. This fat is usually stored as excess fatty tissue or can be specific to the liver. Like excess body fat, fat-soluble vitamins are not removed from the body very easily.

FSVs—vitamins A, D, E, and K—are obtained mostly from fish, red meat, and dairy. Each has specific functions in our bodies:

- *Vitamin A* helps ensure healthy skin, teeth, bones, eyes, and mucus membranes.
- *Vitamin D*, although it is produced in the body, can only be produced when sunlight is absorbed.

Therefore, vitamin D is also known as the sunshine vitamin. Note that normal calcium levels are also important, since vitamin D and calcium work in harmony with each other.

- *Vitamin E* has powerful antioxidants that protect our cells from damage and aging.
- *Vitamin K* is important for clotting and wound healing. It also provides protection to our body tissues and bones. Incidentally, excess vitamin K from a vegetable diet is unknown to cause blood clotting.

WATER-SOLUBLE VITAMINS

Water-soluble vitamins are dissolved by water and absorbed by water. Unlike fat-soluble vitamins, water-soluble vitamins are easily excreted. They assist the body in providing energy to organs and aid in proper nerve function.

There are nine water soluble vitamins:

- B1 (thiamine)
- B2 (riboflavin)
- B3 (niacin)
- B5 (pantothenic acid)
- B6 (pyridoxine)
- B7 (biotin)
- B9 (folate)
- B12 (cobalamin)
- Vitamin C (ascorbic acid)

MINERALS

Minerals are naturally occurring elements obtained from water, plants, and the earth.

Minerals are *not* produced in the body but are highly essential for health and development.

There are more than a dozen essential minerals needed for adequate body function. Some of these are:

- copper
- calcium
- chromium
- chloride
- fluoride
- iron
- magnesium
- potassium
- sulfur
- sodium
- zinc
- iodine

Minerals are obtained from foods such as dark leafy vegetables, shellfish, fruits, nuts, whole grains, avocados, dairy, beans, meats, tofu, and from natural spring and mineral water.

CHAPTER 16

IRON WOMAN

Due to the additional bodily demands women are confronted with, supplemental intake of iron is more prevalent among women as compared to their male counterparts. Iron deficiency (one type of anemia) is more common among women because of the high blood supply required for the menstrual cycle, childbearing, and breastfeeding.

Oxygen is dispersed throughout the human body by means of the hemoglobin molecule in the blood. This hemoglobin molecule is transported by the red blood cells in the blood.

Hemoglobin requires iron, and together they bind to oxygen for delivery to all body cells. Consequently, when iron levels are low, so is the oxygen level. By the way, blood gets its red hue from iron. With low iron (oxygen) come symptoms such as fatigue, anxiety, dizziness, shortness of breath, brittle nails, headaches, compromised immunity, muscle weakness, or restless leg syndrome. Even thyroid dysfunction can result.

Red meat, and animal meat in general, is quite rich in iron, so it's a bit more common for vegetarians to be iron deficient. That said, there are three important tenets to consider. First, plant-based foods do supply adequate iron requirements, but a balanced variety is essential.

Foods such as quinoa, leafy vegetables, peas, beans, soy products, pumpkin seeds, whole grains, pistachios, apricots, prunes, raisins, chocolate, molasses, and others all provide a moderate to high content of iron.

Note that vitamin C or citrus fruits increase the absorption of iron from various plant foods.

Note also that iron supplements should not be taken unless supervised by a physician following a blood test confirmation. A high or excess level of iron is associated with heart disease, insulin-resistant diabetes, and cancer and increases free radicals circulating in the blood.

Lastly, most of the iron in the body is recycled or stored in organs such as the heart, pancreas, and liver. Since there is no regulatory system to eliminate iron from the body, iron overload or toxicity can develop.

CHAPTER 17

GARDEN FRESH

With respect to the buzzwords and understandable pandemonium of the 2020 coronavirus pandemic, I can only speculate that the vegans may well be ahead of the curve.

ADAGES OUR PARENTS MAY HAVE UTTERED

A few of the adages we may have grown up hearing might apply, for example:

- What does not kill fattens. (Esmeralda Santiago)
- Too much of one thing isn't good for nothing. (Ray Bradbury)
- If you do not eat food like medicine, medicine becomes your food. (Hippocrates)
- Eat your vegetables. (anonymous)
- Your body is your temple. (anonymous)

Although these expressions may have slightly different meanings, they all seem to centralize on one subtle but valid point. That is, we must eat sensibly. The term I use is "conscious consumption." This is essentially the antithesis of random or compulsive eating. Throughout this book, I have provided a baseline of information regarding food choices. The idea is to contribute a space of information so that food choices are made from a more informed position.

As a side note, I am blessed to have realized upon learning of the universally appealing superfoods that some of them (soursop, papaya, watercress, purple sweet potatoes, avocados, citrus fruits, bitter melon, and various herbs) were regular staples of my Caribbean upbringing. Incidentally, pineapples, berries, watermelon, cantaloupe, and others all fall under the category of superfoods.

With respect to nutritional value, vegetables speak for themselves. There is no match, as vegetables provide all the essentials and more. Vegetables are part of all the food groups. They furnish all the needed proteins, vitamins, minerals, carbs, water, and fiber, along with the many phytochemicals, antioxidants, flavonoids, and flavones we need.

Although we all know what vegetables are, a list is provided as a reminder of the variety we have available to choose from:

- amaranth greens (taro leaves, a.k.a. callaloo)
- spinach
- bell peppers
- squash
- cucumbers
- cactus leaves
- chard
- sea vegetables (kelp)
- zucchini

- okra
- turnip greens
- beets
- bitter melon
- olives
- bok choy
- avocados
- tomatoes
- onions
- eggplant
- kale
- broccoli
- asparagus
- celery
- collard greens
- pumpkin
- carrots
- cauliflower
- rhubarb
- brussels sprouts
- green papaya
- yellow or purple sweet potatos

Once again, vegetables provide all the minerals, vitamins, and protein we could ever need. They are inexpensive, highly accessible, and provide superior health benefits without the fat or adverse effects of other foods.

CHAPTER 18

COLORFUL SEEDLINGS

39

Fruits are sweet, nutritional, and usually quite cosmetically appealing. While our choices are often selective or limited, consuming a wide variety is highly suggested.

Many of us restrict our taste buds to a half dozen or so variations of fruit. We can consider maximizing our nutritional and antioxidant capacity by devouring a wide range of such delicacies. There are lots of hidden treasures we can select from.

Here are more than thirty fruit choices to contemplate:

- seeded grapes
- pears
- seeded melon
- tamarind
- apples
- apricots
- cantaloupe
- kiwi
- cherries
- persimmons
- papaya
- pomegranate
- limes

- guava
- mangoes
- star fruit
- elderberries
- blueberries
- grapefruit
- breadfruit
- raspberries
- pineapple
- figs
- plums
- honeydew melon
- kumquat
- peaches
- sugar apple
- bananas
- oranges (green and yellow skin)
- ash gourd
- soursop
- ambarella (golden apple, pommecythere)

CHAPTER 19

AT OUR DISPOSAL

Unlike in our current lifestyle, growing up I recall a sense of anticipation—the tease of budding blossoms—as we awaited the explosion of seasonal fruits and vegetables. Aside from several perennials, most of the seventy or so fruits of Trinidad, West Indies, were all seasonally harvested. Weekly visits to the mostly outdoor markets were a visceral sensation as we rummaged through the organized chaos.

By contrast, life in our industrialized countries gives us a very different experience. Although poverty is quite real for a billion of this world's inhabitants, many of us in the modern world are blessed with nonstop quantities of food choices. With technological advancements and the consequential availability of such a wide variety of foods, for many of us, the concept of poverty seems out of sight, out of mind.

As we count our blessings and smell the roses, time breezes by us—to never return. May we become enlightened to the blessings at our disposal and to the needs of others.

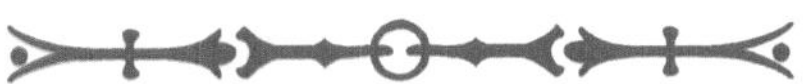

PART III

NUTRITIONAL PEARLS

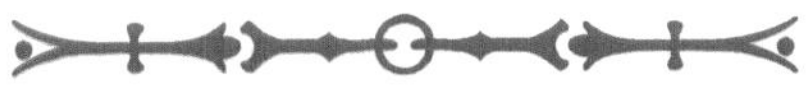

CHAPTER 20

SPECIAL NOTE

45

It seems fair to say that when foods are processed, synthesized, or isolated from their natural state, they often acquire a toxic, addictive, less nutritious, or artificial form. Be it sugar from sugarcane, cocaine from cocoa leaves, asparin from willow bark or starch from wheat barley, the concept applies.

CHAPTER 21

MORNING AROMATICS

B rewed coffee can be thought of as a culture. It is enjoyed by so many of us worldwide. Coffee can be good, bad, or simply a choice.

Caffeinated products (coffee, green tea, energy drinks, soda pop, and eatables) all have similar effects with varying levels of potency or strength. Worldwide, the second most common caffeinated drink is green tea.

Coffee is a central nervous system (brain) stimulant. The hormone adrenaline is released, and dopamine is inhibited. This antagonistic effect provokes the brain and energizes the heart rate. Consequently, you feel good, alert, and energetic but also agitated. Long-term usage (especially if consumed potently, or several cups per day) often results in prolonged adverse effects. Such effects are not limited to accelerated aging appearance, fluid retention, increased blood pressure, lack of natural endurance, and the tendency to become easily angered. In essence, there is conclusive increased stress to the body.

Diarrhea is not uncommon, particularly with occasional users. This is due to the acidic nature and the fiber content of coffee. Why do some of us experience a "crash" several hours after drinking coffee? Well, coffee stimulates the release of a chemical neurotransmitter (hormone) call adenosine. After a duration of time, the caffeine is absorbed (metabolized), while moderate levels of adenosine remain stagnant in the body. This dual effect causes the body to feel tired, sleepy, or lazy.

Hint: Drinking lots of alkaline water aids in reducing such lazy, lethargic feelings.

Some fun facts regarding coffee:

- Ethiopia is known as the original hub for coffee beans.
- The coffee bean is a billion-dollar industry.
- Approximately half the world's population consumes coffee daily.
- Retirees consume the most coffee.
- All commercial coffee is a derivative of two types of coffee. It's either the aromatic, milder "Arabic" form or the inexpensive instant "robust" brand.
- Of the top ten most expensive brews, priced per pound, Jamaican Blue Mountain lands on the bottom at $50 per pound. In contrast, the Kopi Luwak coffee bean ranks at the top for $600 per pound. This Kopi Luwak brew is harvested and fermented via the defecation (stools) of the Asian palm civet—a weasel carnivore.

CHAPTER 22

OILS AND FATS

48

Common use of cooking oils date back to approximately 3000 BC. Such oils were initially introduced by Europeans, and their use was taken up by the Chinese and Japanese about two thousand years ago.

Cooking oil was first obtained from animals and then from plants, and it's now synthetically manufactured. Here are some essential inquiries to consider regarding various cooking oils:

- Is it refined or unrefined?
- What is its boiling point (smoking point)?
- Is it animal or plant based?
- Is it saturated or unsaturated?
- Does it contain trans fat or not?

There are more than two dozen types of oil, so I may fail to mention them all.

Refined oils have a high boiling point (smoking point). This allows the oil to tolerate high heat temperatures before releasing toxic fumes and free radicals. Refined oils are neutral in taste (like most oils) and have an extended shelf life. They are processed through intense heating and bleaching to remove the volatile toxic chemicals. Some common refined oils include vegetable oils (sunflower, corn, and canola) and several others.

Unrefined oils are the cold-pressed, raw, and virgin oils. They are extracted and bottled in their natural state. They are known to be nutritional and flavorful. Olive oil is the classic unrefined oil. However, it has the lowest heating or smoking point at 325 degrees Fahrenheit. This means high heat is not encouraged.

Animal fats are your lards, butter, cheese, and dairy. The key feature here is that animal fats are saturated fatty acids. Saturated fatty acids tolerate intense heat temperatures well. However, they become solids at room temperature. As such, they can remain in the body and cause hardening of the arteries or blood vessel blockage.

This is where trans fats become significant. Trans fat is good for frying and used in most processed and fast foods.

Trans fats are saturated oils. Although they are often used, they provide the most concerns in terms of health. Trans fats are well known for their link to inflammation and heart disease. They are associated with increased LDLs (low density lipoproteins—the bad stuff) in the body.

Just as with most everything in life, oils, too, are about choice. Hopefully, we can make choices that are conscious and informed.

Based on the general information above, here is a sample oil chart to appraise:

Okay	Good	Better
Pork	Grape seed	Extra Virgin
Palm	Sunflower	Organic olive

Coconut	Almond	Flaxseed
Lard	Mustard	Peanut
Butter	Soybean	Avocado
Cotton seed	Canola	Fish oil
Cheese	Canola	Sesame

CHAPTER 23

CREAMY DIARY

51

Although the use of milk dates back to earlier than 10,000 BC in Mesopotamia, daily consumption began at a much later period.

Interestingly enough, this consumption was an evolutionary process. In the earlier days, adults were unable to tolerate or digest milk. They lacked the enzyme lactose, which is needed in order to metabolize milk. Currently about half the world's population is able to digest fresh whole milk.

Products such as kefir, yogurt, and cheese are tolerated by most of the population because the fermentation process breaks down the lactose. Due to this bacterial fermentation breakdown, the lactose enzyme is not demanded for digestion.

MILK

A cup of whole milk contains

- 8 grams of protein,
- 8 grams of fat,
- 150 calories,

- 30 percent of daily recommended allowance of calcium, and
- essential vitamins (B12) and nutrients.

On the flip side, milk ironically extracts calcium from bones. Milk provides saturated (bad) fats. It is typically inundated with secondary antibiotics and hormones from commercial livestock. In addition, milk is also associated with various allergies, acne, and lactose intolerance and is a risk factor for cancer.

Almost two-thirds of all human diseases are attributed to domestication of animals—smallpox, measles, influenza, TB (tuberculosis), and mad cow disease, to name a few.

By the way, hot milk can assist in sound sleep due to the presence of tryptophan, which stimulates serotonin and the sleep hormone called melatonin.

Here are some healthier alternatives to commercial livestock milk:

- oat milk
- cashew milk
- almond milk
- plant-based milk
- rice milk
- quinoa milk
- coconut milk
- soy milk

CHAPTER 24

COCOA CONFECTIONERS

53

The global chocolate industry has an approximate net worth of $100 billion. Two-thirds of all the cocoa is imported from west Africa, with Europe (Switzerland and Germany) leading the world in consumption.

That said, chocolate is risky business for health and nutrition. Yes, dark (100 percent) chocolate cocoa, containing little sugar and no dairy, does provide valuable antioxidants. Polyphenols are the antioxidants, which give the chocolate the bitter taste. Unfortunately, the processed dairy milk in chocolate neutralizes much of the benefits available in these polyphenols.

CHAPTER 25

RED WINE

Resveratrol is known as the healthy antioxidant constituent of red wine. The healthiest choice of the red wines is rumored to be pinot noir. Why? It is said to have the highest concentration of resveratrol, with other red wines in succession. Although red wines all have a low sugar content, Pinot Noirs generally have the lowest residual sugar, furnish the least amount of calories, and contain the least fermented alcohol.

Although Italy, France, and Spain lead the world in production, the United States consumes the most wine.

CHAPTER 26

STARCHES AND GRAINS

Starches and grains provide carbs and energy to the human body. Here are some healthy choices to entertain:

- quinoa
- yams
- green bananas
- wild organic brown rice
- eddoes
- yucca
- potatoes
- spaghetti squash
- nuts
- plantains
- breadfruit (jackfruit family)
- chia
- steel-cut oats
- granola
- rye

CHAPTER 27

CARNIVORE'S DELIGHT

Ironically, in my quest to further understand and learn about the nutritional value of meat,

I am more convinced that a vegetarian diet is unsurpassed by any other dietary lifestyle. In reviewing the pros and cons, there seems to be no sector in which a meat diet lifestyle is superior. At minimum, vegetables provide high levels of antioxidants, are easier to digest, are less expensive, ensure higher nutrient uptake, and are effective in disease prevention.

Nevertheless, it would be unfair to omit a section on our beloved fish and meat dishes. I too have enjoyed eating and, at times, only seemed to be fulfilled when meat was an integral part of my plate. With less than 10 percent of the world population declaring to be vegans/vegetarians, meat is indisputably an entrenched part of our culture and cuisine.

Generally, meat refers to the common domesticated mammals (including birds) that we consume. Red meat, more often than not, is used in reference to beef and pork.

Overall, most of the controversy regarding meat lies with the many toxic chemicals and additives involved in its production. Aside from these noted villains, there are also issues regarding the environmental impact of meat production and consumption.

Nonetheless, there is no debate with respect to the protein and iron that meat provides. In addition to a high volume of protein, meats also supply vitamin B12, iron, zinc, and other nutrients. This is especially significant with farms that employ free-roaming, grass-feeding operations.

Most concerns are geared toward the common practice of GMO livestock. To keep up with demand, it has become imperative for factory farms to widely utilize antibiotics and hormones for the protection and rapid growth of commercial farm animals.

The adverse effects of such wide distribution and usage of chemicals have been passed on to each of us who consume meat and meat products. In short, even though red meats, farm-raised fish, and poultry all provide noteworthy nutritional value, meats also carry the potentially fatal flaw of chemical overuse.

CHAPTER 28

HERBAL TEAS:
A SPICE OF INFORMATION

Unlike the classic green or black caffeinated teas, herbal teas are usually noncaffeinated. The beneficial effects on the human body are well established and without question. Herbal teas are essentially natural plant leaves, seeds, flowers, bark, or fruits. Fortunately, herbs can be used as teas, food supplements, or spices or strictly for medicinal purposes.

For our purpose, herbal teas contribute to improved organ function and disease prevention, as they are crammed with potent antioxidants. Other characteristics drive herbals to be greatly appreciated. Among these, they are

- of infinite variety,
- inexpensive,
- strong immune boosters,
- simply prepared,
- caffeine-free,
- natural,
- easily home grown, and
- interchangeable as seasonings.

Following is a concoction I have been using for the past few years. This herbal mix provides for me a convenient, highly nutritional, long-lasting and delicious hot tea option.

Ingredients

- 1 pound of fresh gingerroot
- 20 heads of clove
- 1 nutmeg
- 10 bay leaves
- 2 tablespoons turmeric powder

1. Wash gingerroots well. You may remove root ends as needed. Cut into small pieces.
2. Place ginger in blender with 1 to 2 cups of water.
3. Blend to liquid puree.
4. Add cloves, grated nutmeg, bay leaves, and turmeric.
5. Mix well with a spoon.
6. Pour into pint-sized containers. Keep one in the refrigerator for daily use. Freeze remaining containers to use as needed.

For a hot cup of tea:

1. Place one teaspoon of ginger mix into tea cup.
2. Add boiling water and enjoy.
3. If needed, add a half teaspoon of honey or your favorite natural sweetener.

Kindly appreciate that herb teas are not rocket science recipes. Unless someone has a very specific objective or issue at hand, any herbal combination from your pantry can work magic. For a cup of tea, I usually mix together a quarter teaspoon of any two herbal spices, add hot water, and savor.

In general, and more so during periods of increased risk of viral infections, hot liquids, such as 2–3 cups of herbal tea each day, can be of great value as a control or preventative measure.

Herbal tea mixtures are simple, nutritious, and cost-effective. The sky is the limit, and you get to own it.

PART IV
SPECIAL CONSIDERATIONS

CHAPTER 29

A WORD OF CONTEMPLATION

To achieve what we want, we must first think it through. Since it is easier to implement a variety of nutritional elements in regard to our physical bodies, usually less emphasis is directed to the optics of our minds. Anything and everything we express, execute, or accomplish is always manifested first in our thoughts. For example, whatever little or however much we gain from reading this book is totally dependent on our mindset. How we think is essentially a reflection of our attitude, our emotions, our memories, and our desires.

Collectively, these features interact to create thoughts. Our thoughts are the precursor to how we feel and how we respond.

Customarily, our thinking is often a knee-jerk, cosmetic reaction, which is swiftly distracted. This seems especially true considering our modern-day, instantly gratifying, high-tech, self-governing lifestyle.

CHAPTER 30

SLEEP DEPRIVATION

Poor sleep habits or inadequate sleep can be quite destructive to the human body. We are familiar with the common signs (moodiness, forgetfulness, anxiety) of inadequate sleep.

These signs and symptoms affect our general health, which in turn effects our life. Stress at some level is usually inevitable. However, when sleep deprivation is compounded with other bodily stresses, the combined effect leads to disease and demise.

We know that sleep deprivation in itself greatly exacerbates any existing stress on the human body. These stress responses can manifest themselves physically or mentally. Physical changes may include the appearance of accelerated aging, clinical ailments, improper digestion, fatigue, weight fluctuations, diminished endurance, and others. Mental stress can be associated with memory loss, mood changes, anxiety, lack of clarity in thought, and even depression.

Melatonin is a chemical substance (hormone) that assists the brain in restoring and regulating the sleep cycle. It is understood to promote sleep and to serve as an essential part of the circadian rhythm. The circadian rhythm is the body's twenty-four-hour time clock, which monitors our sleep/wake cycle. This internal rhythmic mechanism is located in the hypothalamus (deep center) of the brain. It records the sleep cycle of illumination (daybreak) and darkness (nighttime). The melatonin hormone, also of the hypothalamus region, is produced by the pineal gland, which is often referred to as the third eye.

The illustration below is a depiction of the pineal gland in the hypothalamic region of the brain. The brain stem, which is also in this region, extends above the spinal cord. The brain stem is essentially the engine of the human body. It controls our heart rate, breathing, REM sleep, and the responsiveness of our brain itself.

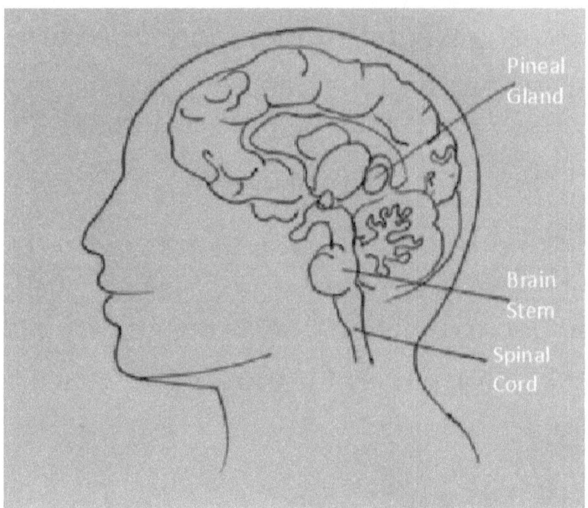

The central point of this information is to convey that health, nutrition, and wellness of the mind and body are pivotal to a healthy, productive life.

CHAPTER 31

INTERMITTENT FASTING

Intermittent fasting is not really a diet or weight-loss program but more of an eating pattern that can be complementary to good health. We typically fast to detox our bodies or as a spiritual custom. Here, we'll focus on intermittent fasting as it applies to well-being.

There appear to be at least three components involved with fasting and weight moderation. They are what you eat, when you eat, and the degree of physical activity you engage in.

Note: Eating to capacity or in excess is also a component but not discussed in this text.

Note: Due to the nature of the disease, fasting is not recommended to individuals diagnosed with diabetes.

First, what you eat is of utmost importance. Let's look at the diagram below.

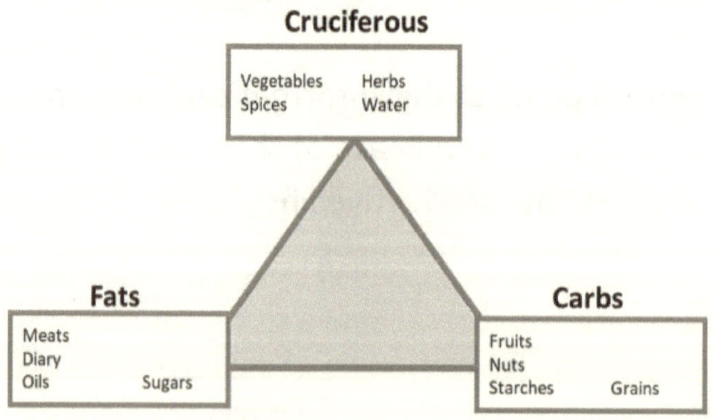

If we consume primarily cruciferous foods, we acquire good nutrition and no fats.

When we add carbs, we obtain good nutrition, extra energy, and some fats.

If we also consume fats, we receive all of the above plus possible weight gain.

The second component is food timing. Food takes roughly one to three hours to digest depending on the food type and your metabolic rate.

A rewarding fast may require at least twelve hours of zero food intake. This can be accomplished most trouble free during sleep or nighttime. If we include three hours for food digestion, we would need to eat our last meal fifteen hours before breakfast. For example, we can have dinner at 7:00 p.m., allow three hours for digestion (now 10 p.m.), and then break our fast at 10:00 a.m. This allows for the body to utilize all its nutrient energy. In the interim, we are able to optimize the digestion and absorption of our food.

Furthermore, the body is able to more efficiently cleanse and detox itself.

The third component is physical activity. With a specific cardio-physical exercise routine, fat utilization can be accomplished. Ultimately, with an understanding of all constituents, we should not have to starve ourselves or invoke unnecessary risk to our bodies to enjoy the benefits of intermittent fasting.

CHAPTER 32

YOGA NAMASTE

Particularly in the Western world, yoga, similar to martial arts, is often practiced as a fad or just another thing to do. However, historically and with its true purpose, yoga is a deeply spiritual, mental, and physical discipline.

The teachings and philosophy of yoga, in themselves, help to guide the practitioner toward a more purposeful life. It helps us to embrace the fact that there is so much that we don't know when compared to that we do know. I believe this is significant and applicable on any level.

Maturing to such awareness allows us to be attentive, humble, and open to all thoughts and ideas. There is also an inherent peace and inner delight that comes with such mindfulness.

According to historical records, yoga has been around for more than five thousand years. The terms *yoga* and *mantra* (along with yoga's rituals and sacred history) were first noted in ancient texts of India referred to as the Vedas. Shiva is the god of yoga. Ayurveda essentially incorporates herbal treatments alongside the health and well-being of yoga practices. Yoga is described as a connection or balance between mind and body. It is essentially a spiritual discipline with lots of perks. The practice of yoga induces physical strength, flexibility, a sense of discipline, deep breathing respiratory exercises, meditation, health awareness, self-realization, and ultimately a oneness between mind and body. In essence, yoga provides for a higher form of physical and mental consciousness.

Among the numerous styles and forms of yoga, one personal favorite yoga practice involves a variety of breathing exercises. These breathing techniques are known to provide incredible health (respiratory and circulatory) benefits.

In the process, increased mental clarity, inner joy, increased lung capacity, attenuation of snoring and deep relaxation are gained.

There are many occasions when we feel truly elated, relaxed, or enlightened. Such moments of bliss can be experienced when we are well rested and stress free; when we're in peaceful places, such as at the beach; when experiencing financial rewards, deep gratitude, or liberation; when we're "in love," during intimacy, when observing our new baby; in the course of prayer, and during a born-again Christian experience, to name a few.

There is no doubt that the discipline of yoga (physical well-being, nutrition, and meditative practices) can capture a similar euphoric state.

I call this space of exhilaration "my positive domain."

CHAPTER 33

EXERCISE ROUTINE

As we all know, physical exercise has proven to be extremely valuable for the proper functioning of every cell and organ of the human body. Physical activity can improve mind-body health in at least two fundamental ways. The first is cardiovascular (heart and blood circulation) improvement. With increased strength and function of the heart, optimum blood circulation of oxygen and food nutrients enable them to be optimally absorbed into the body cells. This is why you feel rejuvenated after physical exercise.

Among other benefits, exercise tends to lower our blood pressure, which is directly related to a more robust longevity.

The second considerable reward to physical exercise is attributed to increased muscle, improved tone, and a rise in flexibility. This translates to long-standing personal independence during life.

Although in the course of exercising, there is inevitable micromuscle damage, fortunately, there is also critical rebuilding and recovery of body muscle after exercise. One key factor in maximizing your cardiovascular and muscle strength lies with incorporating adequate fluids and nutritional intake. Sufficient rest and sleep are also quite significant.

As you have observed, only a few gains are outlined in this topic on exercise. Efficient elimination of body waste (our next topic) is just one of many such gains. There are numerous additional benefits to a comprehensive, cardio-physical workout.

As we try to enhance the physical body, may we also enhance the physical geometry of life. And may we remember that all of such gains are most rewarding and guarded when accomplished during a pleasant state of mind.

CHAPTER 34

FOOD ELIMINATION

On a whole, there is no normal number of times a day a person should have a bowel movement. Some people poop once daily, while others engage five times a day. Providing there are no persistent, unchanging bloody, black, or watery stools, the frequency of poops is usually arbitrary. Generally speaking, stools (poop) can also be any color, depending on your diet and the type of foods you eat.

However, it is a healthier practice to have your colon (large intestine, which stores your poop) emptied frequently. An empty colon means there is far less unnecessary waste and toxic accumulation in your body.

General waste elimination takes shape in many forms and outlets. There are liquids, solids, and gases to be removed from the body. The various human organs that are involved include the kidneys, eyes, stomach, lungs, sweat glands, nostrils, rectum, skin, ears, and oral cavity. Collectively, these organs often eliminate the equivalent of 6–8 glasses of liquid daily. Hence, the recommendation of replenishing the body with several glasses of water each day.

Although foodstuff is often not eliminated from the body until twelve to twenty-four hours after it is consumed, stomach digestion requires a shorter time span. Specifically:

- Water takes a couple of minutes.
- Fruits and veggies take roughly forty-five minutes.
- Seafood usually requires at least an hour.
- Starches, chicken, and milk take more or less two hours.
- Red meat, nuts, and grains demand at least three hours

Water, exercise, and a diet high in fiber help to bulk and eliminate foods at ease.

Here is a list of high-fiber foods:

- coffee
- papaya
- citrus
- spinach
- broccoli
- prunes
- apple juice
- rye bread
- avocado
- kefir milk
- rhubarb plant (contains senna)
- sweet potatoes (yellow and purple)
- pears
- figs
- artichokes
- beans

PART V

ORGAN-SPECIFIC FOOD COMPLEMENTS

CHAPTER 35

A COMMENTARY OF REITERATION

The information presented throughout this text basically touches the surface of various wellness-related subjects. This concise approach, as opposed to one that's inundated with information difficult both to process and retain, can be both rewarding and liberating. My intent is to introduce established and individual information for inspiration, further inquiry, and personal empowerment.

The upcoming topic may be considered the least favorable by some. For others, it may be the most valued. One reason some may shy away from pairing specific foods with specific organ health is that all fresh organic fruits, herbs, and vegetables provide a major source of nutrition and defense for the entire human body. With a balanced (highly inclusive) consumption of natural foods, all body organs are inherently fortified. Secondly, while there is no doubt that specific foods are good for specific organs (this is verifiable), there is always much more involved than what a list can provide.

In any event, the remainder of this chapter lists foods that are most beneficial to specific organs of the human body by organ.

EYES

- carrots
- dandelions
- carrot greens
- bok choy
- water
- red and yellow bell peppers
- cruciferous vegetables

BLOOD AND BLOOD VESSELS

- sarsaparilla
- grapes
- water
- cumin
- coriander
- bitter foods
- cruciferous vegetables

LIVER

- beets
- spinach
- broccoli
- citrus
- turmeric
- avocado
- garlic

- kale
- pure cocoa
- cinnamon
- cruciferous vegetables
- arugula
- water
- basil
- apples

HEART

- pure cocoa
- carrots
- oranges
- beets
- kale
- blueberries
- water
- cruciferous vegetables

KIDNEYS

- cranberries
- blueberries
- water
- cardamom
- herbs
- cruciferous vegetables

GI TRACT

- cumin
- coriander
- cardamom
- cranberries
- dandelion
- cruciferous vegetables
- fever grass
- cinnamon
- water
- pineapple

IMMUNE SYSTEM

- fever grass
- basil
- pineapple
- garlic
- oregano
- onions
- water
- cruciferous
- habanero peppers
- radishes
- turmeric
- honey
- citrus
- echinacea
- cruciferous vegetables

RESPIRATORY SYSTEM

- citrus
- ginger
- turmeric
- thyme
- honey
- pineapple
- horseradish
- berries
- broccoli
- garlic
- cruciferous vegetables

BRAIN AND NERVES (CENTRAL NERVOUS SYSTEM)

- avocado
- banana
- blueberries
- beets
- pomegranate
- olive oil
- rosemary
- pure cocoa
- ginger
- sage
- turmeric
- soursop
- spinach
- chamomile

- oatmeal
- broccoli
- taro leaves
- salmon
- walnuts
- pumpkin
- cinnamon
- whole grains
- sardines
- almond
- cruciferous vegetables
- pumpkin seeds

SKIN

The skin is the largest organ in the body. Here are some nutritionally rich foods specific to good skin health:

- all berries
- fatty fish
- walnuts
- sunflower seeds
- dark pure chocolate
- red grapes
- cruciferous vegetables
- kiwi
- guava
- sweet potato

- avocado
- soy
- broccoli
- water

CHAPTER 36

CRUCIFEROUS VEGETABLES

84

Cruciferous vegetables can be thought of as super nutrient-rich vegetables, whereby many of the flowers, leaves, and even the roots are edible.

They include arugula, kale, broccoli, turnips, watercress, collard greens, radishes, brussels sprouts, cabbages, sweet potatoes, bok choy, spinach, carrots, and others.

PART VI
CLINICAL CORNER

CHAPTER 37

HALF EMPTY, HALF FULL

No doubt, this protracted, unpredictable, and tragic period of the 2020 coronavirus will be remembered for some time to come. Respect and homage to the many lives directly impacted and those who have, sadly, demised.

Notwithstanding, I am more convinced that much good will be wrenched from this experience. It already appears that more of the world is increasingly diligent and appreciative of family, health, joy, and Mother Nature, as well as the simple novelties of life. To this end, I am truly thankful.

CHAPTER 38

HOW THE EYES SEE

How the eyes function is often compared to the way a camera works. The retina is like the film. The image we see is composed of light, which is reflected from the object. Reflections from objects enter the eye and then go to the brain for interpretation. Please see figure 47.1.

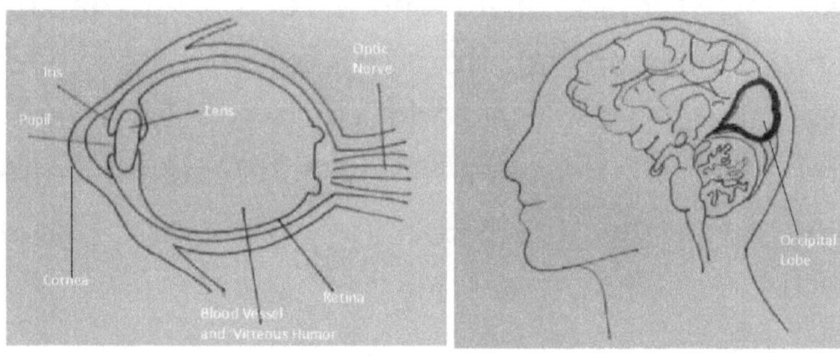

Figure 47.1. Cornea ➔ Iris ➔ Pupils ➔ Lens ➔ Retina ➔ Optic Nerve ➔ Brain

To shed some light, light first enters the cornea. Next, it travels to the pupil and then to the lens and, subsequently, to the retina. The image in the retina is inverted due to the slanted anatomy of the eye as light passes through. Photo receptors (sensor cells) in the retina turn this light into electrical signals, which then travel to the optic nerve. Signals from the optic nerve proceed directly to the occipital lobe of the brain for interpretation.

The occipital lobe of the brain is located in the back of the head and is associated with vision and balance. This occipital lobe receives signals from the optic nerve and turns these signals into right-side-up images. Finally, a person's memory works in harmony with his or her five senses to encode, store, or retrieve such information.

The most important organ of all the sensory organs is believed to be the eye. As you know, there are five senses, which are seeing, hearing, touching, tasting, and smelling. Why is seeing so valued?

Approximately 80 percent of all the information we internalize is learned through sight. Comparatively, approximately 50 percent of the information we hear is retained.

Do the following ideas seem familiar?

- Do as I do (what you see), not as I say.
- "I saw" is more convincing than "I heard."
- Seeing is believing.
- Hearsay is nowhere near as strong as "I saw."

All of these notions point to the fact that seeing is the ultimate of the senses.

Thankfully, for unsighted individuals, all other senses become far more heightened and powerful.

Rods are a few specialized cells located in the retinal area of the eye. They are linked to night vision. Cones are an abundance of cells located in the fovea and the retina area. Cones are associated with daytime (sharp) vision.

Here are some common ailments related to the eye:

- Pink eye. Inflammation of the eyelid.
- Cataracts. Cloudy lens, which is age related.
- Glaucoma. Optic nerve damage due to increase pressure of the eyeball. Glaucoma is usually treated, not cured.
- Keratoconus. Corneal bulging and thinning caused by insufficient protective antioxidants of the cornea.
- Diabetic retinopathy. Blood vessel damage to the retina.
- Dryness. Inadequate lubrication or tears. Tears are a combination of mucus, water, and fats.
- Macular degeneration. The loss of vision at the center of the eye. Macular degeneration can be caused by fatty deposits under the retina or leaky blood vessels.

Vitamin A and beta-carotene keep the surface of the eye moist and healthy. Oranges and other colorful fruits and vegetables are all rich in carotene and other vitamins needed for good sight.

CHAPTER 39

DOCTOR'S VISIT

Can nutrition and wellness of the mind and body be metaphorically disconnected upon visiting your medical doctor for an annual checkup? Here is a far-reaching example.

Upon your visit to see your doctor, an electrocardiogram (EKG OR ECG) is initiated. The electromechanical results are printed, and the findings are interpreted. The diagnose is then made, and you are offered a prescription medication for treatment. One question often not considered is, What is the mind-body source of the illness or condition? What might be the root cause? Placing trauma and infectious diseases on the sidelines, the underlying cause of most illnesses are related to a physical, mental, or nutritional imbalance. Most related illnesses can be treated and/or avoided with physical health, holistic nutrition, and nonprescription therapeutics.

However, holistic medicine is not widely in use in modern medical care for several reasons. A few of the reasons and rationales for this include

- the economic pharmaceutical monopoly,
- limited research and clinical trials,

- lack of dosage specificity, and
- inadequate reproducibility and reliability.

This information is not to assert that modern medicine is not superior or that holistic herbal medicine is not of equal value.

CHAPTER 40

CANCEL CANCER

Although cancer itself compromises the immune system, most traditional cancer treatments further weaken the immune system. Cancer is an abnormal cell growth. Cells basically go haywire. Anticancer drugs try to stop this abnormal cell growth. This is done by implementing drugs or radiation that can destroy this abnormal cell growth at its reproductive site.

Normally, the immune system fights infections, inflammation, and diseases of the body. When cancer cells invade the body, the immune system becomes ineffective in fighting the cancer. Anticancer medications are given in an attempt to destroy the cancer cells. In so doing, the immune system is unfortunately and inevitably shattered. Fortunately, in certain variations of cancer, immunotherapy is administered. This approach attempts to strengthen the existing immune system.

Some individuals may have a genetic factor or predisposition for cancer. Even so, in most cancer cases, lifestyle or environmental risk factors usually trigger the onset of the disease.

Life is to be enjoyed, for stress is the intangible nucleus of cancer.

CHAPTER 41

SUGAR DIABETES

As a post type 2 diabetic, I am pleased to attest that a comprehensive nutritional (holistic) lifestyle can be highly effective in normalizing type 2 diabetes.

In general, the primary risk factors for diabetes include a family history, alcohol, overweight, high fatty acids, high blood pressure, and others.

Of the three macro nutrients (protein, fiber and carbohydrates) in our daily diet, carbs are the primary contributors to high blood sugar levels in diabetes. In our bodies, carbs are broken down to sugars for the purpose of energy and storage. The pancreas (a body organ) secretes a hormone called insulin so that sugars leave the blood and enter into the various body cells.

CARBS

What exactly are carbohydrates (carbs)?

The basic food groups are water, minerals, vitamins, vegetables, fiber, protein, fats, and carbs. Carbs are your sugars, starches, dairy, grains, and fruits. Carbs provide most of the glucose in our blood. Carbs also provide most of the fuel energy we utilize each day. There are good (low carb) and bad (high carb) foods.

Fats can also provide carbs and lots of stored energy,

along with drawbacks when not utilized. Fat disrupts cells' ability to absorb insulin. Consequently, high or uncontrolled blood sugar levels are experienced.

Type 1 diabetes is an autoimmune (naturally occurring against itself) disease process. Here, the cells of the pancreatic organ, which produces the insulin hormone, is destroyed. With the insulin-producing cells of the pancreas all destroyed, there is no insulin circulating to trigger the blood sugar to enter the cells. Consequently, sugar accumulates in the blood. And so you have high blood glucose or type 1 diabetes. Although nutritional and lifestyle changes can be effective, insulin therapy is usually inevitable.

In *type 2* diabetes, the pancreas, along with its insulin-producing cells, are normal. However, the receptors (beta sensors) of the body cells are malfunctioning. The body cells can't recognize the insulin, so the cells don't absorb the insulin. Consequently, the sugar in the blood isn't absorbed, and high blood glucose is experienced.

In both type 1 and type 2 diabetes, insulin is the culprit and high sugar in the blood is the disease. Unlike type 1, type 2 diabetes is often reversible with attentive lifestyle changes.

PART VII

A LITERARY ADJOURNMENT

CHAPTER 42

A PAUSE BEFORE NEW POSSIBILITIES

If I may, let's take a pause or time out, as we have just blown through countless subtopics on health and nutrition.

During the next two parts—"Food for Thought" and "Fruit for Thought"—we'll touch and expound on a few of life's more delicate subjects. Some of the narratives, quotes, expressions, and poetic recitals included in these parts may, at times, seem a bit pungent.

Nevertheless, my soul's intent is fashioned toward well-being—a pleasant state of mind and life in itself. The idea is not to persuade but to engage or entertain thoughts from a differing and relaxed voice.

Invariably, we are highly likely to encounter most of the life situations addressed. It is my hope that, upon such engagement, our minds will be receptive to new possibilities.

PART VIII

FOOD FOR THOUGHT

CHAPTER 43

BODY-BASED WELLNESS

The subject of intimacy, health, and relationships may have a wide variety of implications. My focus is briefly directed toward nutritional sustenance and mind-body wellness.

Although everyone is likely to have unique and interesting experiences, a few fundamentals appear to be universal. Our mindset, our physical health, our measure of stability, and our emotional attraction seem to resonate as cornerstones of body-based wellness. Our emotions and responsiveness also play supportive roles.

CHAPTER 44

GEMS OF INTIMACY

Healthy body-based relationships are constructs of appreciation and need. When there is no appreciation and no need, relationships usually dissolve. *The gems of intimacy* is a concept created to illustrate the treasures of intimacy, endurance, and admiration in relationships—with gemstones as an analogy used to build a model relationship.

Sapphires represent the ultimate in a relationship—the foundation—the virtue of being a loving person to another and to oneself. Sapphires represent the point when exuberance is unyielding and a healthy mindset is harmonized. This blissful experience in a relationship is often described as infatuation, being in love, falling head over heels, being on fire, feeling in sync, a magical connection, love at first sight, meeting a knight in shining armor, or just good chemistry.

For a developing relationship to be sustained at any level of significance, other essentials become inescapable. Communication, caring, compromise, commitment, growth, and respect allow for the blossoms of a lasting relationship to be realized.

Emeralds can be viewed as your physical health and wellness. Being nutritionally fortified and physically fit as a lifestyle speaks volumes. This holistic practice provides immeasurable rewards to self and to a body-based relationship.

Health and independence are supreme—and this applies to a union between people. When the body is functioning smoothly, the union is less stressed and more exalted. There are obvious limitations and special circumstances that arise over time.

However, the commitment to endure sets the tone for a purposeful relationship. Incorporating the various nutritional tenets mentioned throughout this book, should contribute to a strong somatic union.

Pearls are the enhancements. These enhancements can be personal, financial, or otherwise. With respect to economics, financial stability is truly wonderful when possible. Should this not be the case, two features can allow this position to be far less worrisome. The first aim is to maintain and cultivate the gems of the sapphire and emerald. The second objective is to deeply understand and embrace the fact that less can be more. With good health and each other, the sky is your limit. Health is your wealth, attitude is everything, and keeping up with the Joneses is pointless.

CHAPTER 45

ANECDOTAL HERBAL ENHANCEMENTS

For completeness and reading entertainment, I would like to touch on the subject of herbal enhancements or aphrodisiacs. As popular as they seem to be, there is little research or evidence-based medicine to substantiate their effectiveness. The support for these mostly plant-based remedies is strictly anecdotal, and no scientific proof can substantiate their efficacy or regulate their dosages.

A handful of these herbal libido supplements include:

- yohimbe
- pure cocoa
- saffron
- ginkgo biloba
- ginseng
- maca sweet roots
- raw oysters
- pistachio nuts
- omega fatty acids
- sea moss (Irish moss)
- tongkat ali extract
- chili peppers

- bois
- banda bark
- tribulus terrestris herbs (puncture vine)
- horny goat weed (*Epimedium*)

In conclusion, one may ask, Why are these supplements relatively popular when in fact the scientific community generally disregards them? In short, aphrodisiacs do serve as a contributory arousal stimulant. This is because of their aromatics, antioxidants, physical configurations, masochistic sensations, hormonally relaxing, and blood circulatory increasing properties. They can relax the mind, stimulate the heart, or amplify the senses. However, inappropriate usage can lead to potential bodily risk.

PART IX

FRUIT FOR THOUGHT

CHAPTER 46

FROM THE HEART

While we may often say the phrase, "I know," in order to express that we understand and are open to new perspectives, we are obliged to prune that notion.

LIFE DEFINED

Love divine
Good and evil
Word of God
Body and mind
Birth and death
Flesh and blood
Fun and games
Faith and grace
Time and energy
Carbon atoms
The Holy Spirit
Chaos and order
God's creation
Mother Nature
Organic matter
A natural force
Forms of energy
A state of being
The supernatural
Balance and infinity
A moment in time

That which we live
Health and wellness
Spirit consciousness
Change and liberation
What you make of it
The present moment
God's image in action
Elements in harmony
The peak of existence
Movement and growth
Response and purpose
Cosmos and the present
Memory and expressions
Choices and experiences
Beauty and thankfulness
Consciousness and desire
Capacity and fulfillment
Reproduction and change
Vibrations and waveforms
Memory and consciousness
The known and the unknown
A microcosm of the universe
Water, earth, fire, air, heavens
Bearers of feminine principle
Dimensions and reverberations
Choice between bliss and agony
Beyond meaning and beyond disclosure

———

The care we take, the attitudes we adopt, and the choices we make govern the magnitude of our lives.

CHAPTER 47

NUANCED QUOTES

Your thoughts may guide your actions
But your emotions guide your attitude.

Do less for more;
Let respect be the lead,
Plan be the purpose,
Values be the goal.

Speak less of others' shortcomings;
It's for your improvement also.

The thought is likened to the rhetoric;
The meaning is likened to the response.
Selfishness I'm opposed to,
Yet I give my all
To those who are appreciative.

Sweet and sour are the fruits of
Our consciousness,
Our labor, and
Our dreams.

Smiles soothe our souls like infectious symbols of love.

Respond with appreciation so that others receive less pain.

At times, one may wonder, Has the bridge of Patriotism
    traversed from
Inclusiveness,
Civil duties,
And respect
To individualism, post-truth, and divisiveness?

Our potential is always greater than the construct of
    our challenge.

Enjoy every interval of life
So that you are winning at every moment.

Freedom is likened to order and regulations,
As autocracy is to chaos and boundlessness.

Every successful feat necessitates a work of diligence and
    a mind of silver linings.

Are we most prone to liking someone who is successful or
    liking someone who succeeds at appreciating?

A simplistic lifestyle is apt to produce an enriched household.

Isn't it precious to be respectfully authentic with an
    unyielding capacity for empathy and thankfulness?

Marriage—half challenge, half luxury,
All good.

Decisions are choices.
Choices shape our destiny.

Mortality is an unpredictable inevitability,
But a legacy can keep your name alive.

Welcome,
As what was acceptable then is now ludicrous
And what was unbearable is now fashionable.

Quietly enjoy the moment, for in that solitude,
Comes inspiration.

Respect is "character beyond measure," while appreciation
   is an inner desire

Love is an action word. By itself, it has no meaning.

Contentment, compassion, and truth are Soulful virtues
   of liberation.

CHAPTER 48

NARRATIVES, EXPRESSIONS AND POETIC RHYTHMS

*J*oy, *peace*, and *happiness* can be fully experienced as one exudes exuberance, compassion, and a pleasant state of mind. Therefore, it is not something we should seek after but something we become.

We talk about unity, one race, bipartisanship, equality, and the like. Yet we are very deeply rooted, with stems antithetical to what we speak.

Meditation may help to clear our minds and stimulate new thoughts, while aiding us to clearly disengage from the contamination of shortsighted thinking.

Should the tag of "immigrant" be expunged from the lexicon?

Possibilities are visualized when positivity is realized.

The only problems there really are lie within the confines of oneself.

Ultimately, time is relevant to each hour, as we are ever closer to our state of demise. Enjoy.

COMPLEXION: A PROPOSAL FOR A LEXICON UPGRADE

This thought may seem far-fetched within the confines of this book. However, a positive definition for a word can, in itself, reduce apprehension and go a long way toward greater unification and wellness of a people.

For a greater state of balance, the proposed word to receive an upgraded definition is "black."

Neither black nor white are true colors, yet they are shades of the same waveform. The lexicon, along with all variations of word finders, could modernize the definition of "black." May it be represented in the same positive, glorious light as the word "white." Such lexicon upgrade is an attempt to further unite humanity by ensuring we view these two words—"black" and "white"—as complimentary, distinguished, and coexisting words of honor.

Fortunately, half the work is done, as the word "white," from its genesis, has already acquired a pedestal—a position of positivity and pleasantness on a global front.

May we now suggest a definition for the word "black":

> Amalgamated in the continent of Africa, descendants of all corners of the earth.
>
> Able to exist in nature without light; natural beauty; strong; majestic; resilient; brilliant.
>
> Afrocentric; describing those believed to be the first Homo sapiens on earth; representative of the motherland, mother of humankind; a spiritually soulful people; trendy; descendants of royalty; believed to

be the oldest word of an indigenous genesis; relating to land of the Kemetic people— Moors, Ethiopians, Egyptians, Nubians; a people of color.

Inclusive; tolerant; absorbs all colors of the visible spectrum of light.

A complexion of the human race; historically powerful; "sun" protected; dark; tan.

Artfully talented; resembling coffee, chocolate, tea; evoking elegance, mystery.

To glaze; to burn; to shine.

Harmonious with Mother Nature.

Athletically inclined.

Representative of mourning; darkness; demise.

Melanin enhanced; an enslaved people; most exploited yet envied and denounced of a people.

According to historian and author Charles Henderson, "In Christian Symbolism, it [black] denotes Holy Spirit. It's the color of Pentecost, said to represent the absolute, constancy, eternity, or the womb ... Black is the liturgical color of Good Friday."

May this proposed upgrade provide an "inertia for balance" within the defined shades of humankind.

LIFE

We are but a speck,
Even less significant than an ant,
Wholly dependent.
From when are oxygen, electricity, and thought derived?

WHAT WE KNOW

Upon realization that, for each of us, our level of ignorance
    far surpasses what we know,
Only then,
May we understand and be receptive to the discernment
    of politics, religion, cultural ethnicities, and life itself
    with unselfish responsiveness.

PARADISE

Streets of gold, angels, comfort, life on earth, a glimmer
of hope, cosmos, spirit consciousness, immortality, faith,
a vault of the unknown, heaven, the saved, the divine, the
choice within us, inner blissfulness, the abode of God.

RELIGION

An institutional, ubiquitous grounding of beliefs, governed
to incite an appreciation for pearls of reverence, often with
an unbroadened perspective.

KNOWLEDGE

Knowledge is rarely new, but the timing, the deliverer, and how the information is perceived dictate its value.

MEN

Physical sexual kings, inclined to latent maturity and apt to express love through accomplishments, gifts, and security.

WOMEN

Beautiful, emotional queens, endowed with the capacity to love, reproduce, and nourish; microcosms of ambivalence who expresses love through words, touch, and body language.

TRIAD OF WELL-BEING

Spiritual—Enlightenment
Physical—Health
Cognitive—Memory and possibilities

WHO AM I

Born and raised a Catholic,Grew up among Hindus A grandson of an East Indian.
Married a queen allied to Seventh-day Adventists.
Accepted Jesus in the Church of Christ
Entrenched nondenominational Baptist.
Appreciator of the philosophy of Buddhism.
Believer in the power of prayer.
An offspring of the African diaspora.
Seeker of growth, learning, and inspiration.
A veteran American.
A child of God.
An advocate for inclusiveness.
Lover of country music.
An ordinary man.

MARRIAGE

The amalgamation of two individuals—
Independent minds,
Independent bodies,
Independent needs—
In love.
Ascends to the bond of endearment—
The chemistry of ecstasy
Hormonal zealousness
Unyielding potential—
All realized

As love takes refuge, only to blossom with bliss
Once again.

DISCIPLINE

Discipline does not imply that we should refrain from indulging
but that we do so with caution, intent, and responsibility.

THINK MORTALITY

As the irrefutable finiteness of life
Becomes alive,
The potential for the beauty of life's purpose
Becomes infinite.

TRUTH

The gospel truth,
The pinnacle of godliness
Inner liberation
Your perception
The space between compassion and character
Accepted facts
The now.

INTELLIGENCE

Experience, knowledge, and understanding,

conveyed with clarity, often without absolutes, and escorted with an open ear for more.

ANXIETY

The source of all stress materializes when things don't go our way. Likewise, when things don't go our way, blossoms of opportunity come our way. The key differentiation between these two parallels lies with our frame of mind.

IGNORANCE

Thinking that you "already know" or failing to understand what you don't know are fundamental inhibitors to further insight.

A DICHOTOMY OF WHAT IF

What if I am a Christian or not?
Should I "speak out" or not?

What if it's regarding the right to bear ... Regulations feared?
Should I or not?

What if it addresses an all-inclusive history/patriotism?
Should I or not?

What if it involves brutality/justice?
Should I or not?

What if it's in respect to the right to choose / due process
of life?
Should I or not?

What if it's about orientation/favoritism?
Should I or not?

What if it's in reference to inequality / racial reckoning?
Should I or not?

What if it concerns the unfitness/excellence of our top
leadership?
Should I or not?

What if it's about the decency of a person who subscribes
to the opposing political party?
Should I or not?

What if it's about biased news reinforced by my favorite
news media outlet?
Should I or not?

What if I am not personally adversely effected?
Should I or not?

Speaking up or silence—this is frequently a "nitpicking
choice," contingent upon:
Personal experience;
Upbringing;

Feelings;
Shortsightedness;
Political affiliation;
Religion;
Favorite news media;
How informed, diverse, and understanding one's
    perspective is;
Who is adversely affected;
Whether information is factual versus opinionated;
My insignificant biased self, and
The question remains:

What if?

INTENTION

Intention may be the ultimate distinction between doing wrong, doing right, or simply not doing.

As you know, politics is a fierce and complex theme, irrespective of one's moral compass. Our position (mindset) is likely to be predicated on our experience, source of information, and intent. Attempting to persuade someone during an initial discourse or debate is likely to be futile or fatal.

One possible resolve is to take a step back. If I align myself with an open ear to learn, understand, and cognitively welcome the convictions of the contrasting view, we become better positioned to rise to a higher level. This approach, though time-consuming, creates a sense of trust, respect, and hope.

Mortality is ahead of us all, and the issue should not be about my position. Instead, the objective can be about balance, understanding, and that new possibilities can become a reality for the good of us all.

In essence, who's right or wrong may be irrelevant, as parallel thinking is unlikely to unite. It's all about igniting change for enlightenment.

What if we internally cultivate and externally exude a pleasant state of being coequally?

We are, perhaps, inherently impregnated with a sinful nature. But we are universally engulfed with unconscious love. Embrace the moment.

CONCLUSION

Allow me to express my heartfelt thanks, as this narrative took shape through personal interest and a desire to share. It is my hope that this book provides some level of ease, inspiration, and information as we inch closer to a balanced state of well-being.

Life is about growth, enjoyment, experiences, and enlightenment—each in our own special way. The consciousness of enjoying each day and, if possible, each hour, is a worthy challenge as we search for that "nugget of good" in each encounter. Different experiences may necessitate letting go, being involved, or just being amenable to new possibilities.

Enlightenment implies a higher level of consciousness. It involves thinking and relating a little beyond the everyday madness, materialism, and media frenzy.

Constituents of cognitive enrichment (the mind) incorporate gratitude, generosity, meditation, fresh air, sunshine, challenges, restfulness, faith, and objective thinking, along with physical and nutritional health.

Finally, I would like to address the challenge of stress reduction. This instinctive, exploitive etiquette or behavior is difficult to dodge. Stress reduction can be attained through the practice of yoga, laughter, a walk to the park, a cell phone "getaway," musings, and much more. Included is a vital, conscious awareness that life events are *not* going to go our way every day.

It is my hope that we all can take a moment to reflect, appreciate, and engage our minds and bodies—moving toward a life of good health, nutrition, and wellness.

———

For each hour that breezes by, we are ever so much closer to the mortality of life.
Enjoy.

PHOTO GALLERY

129

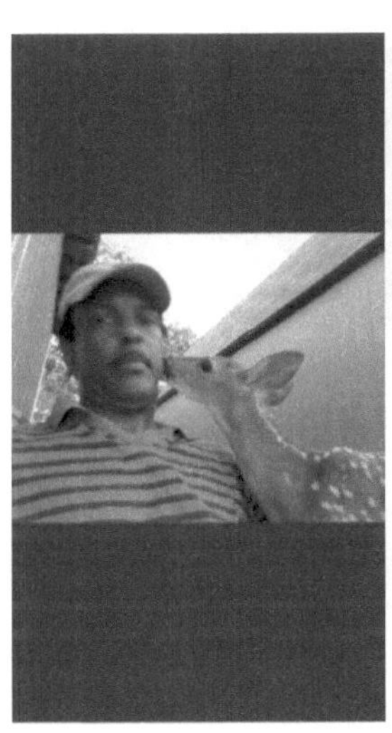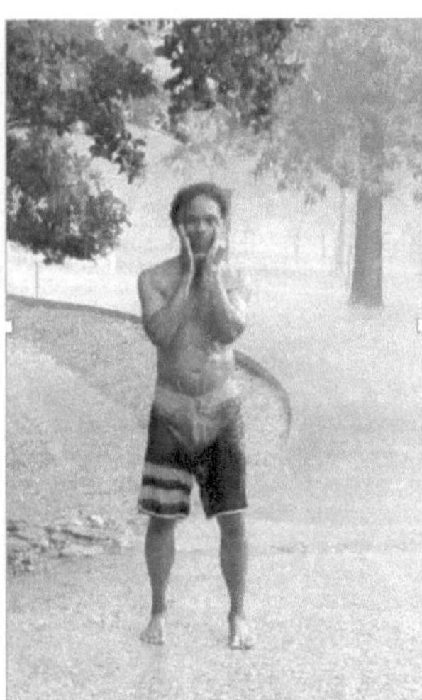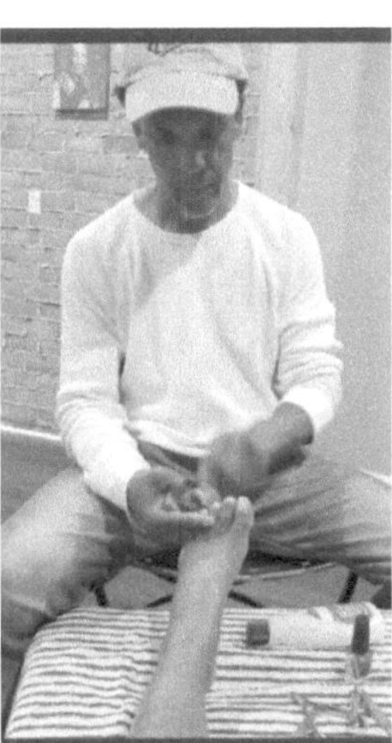

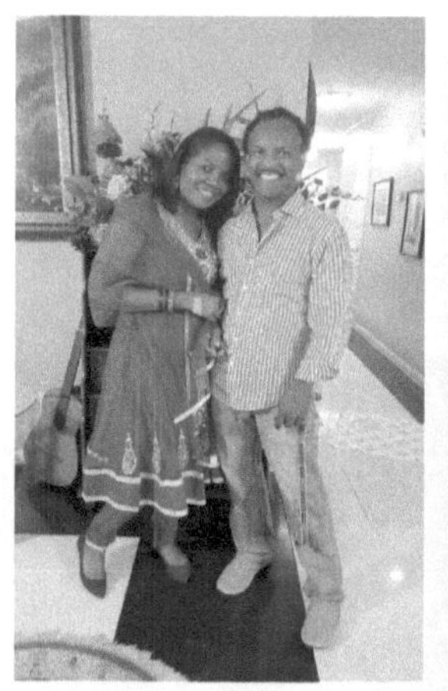

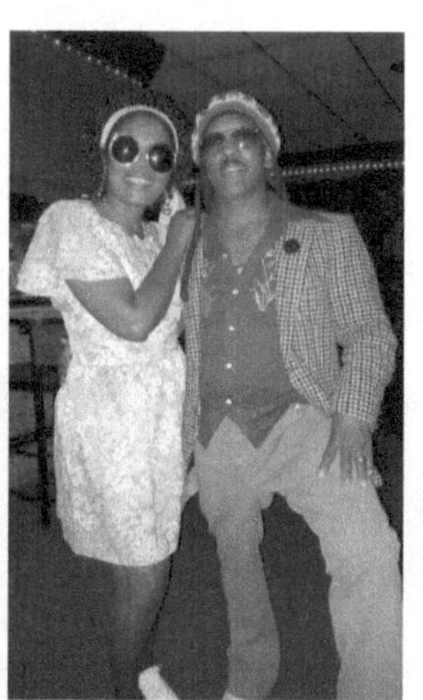

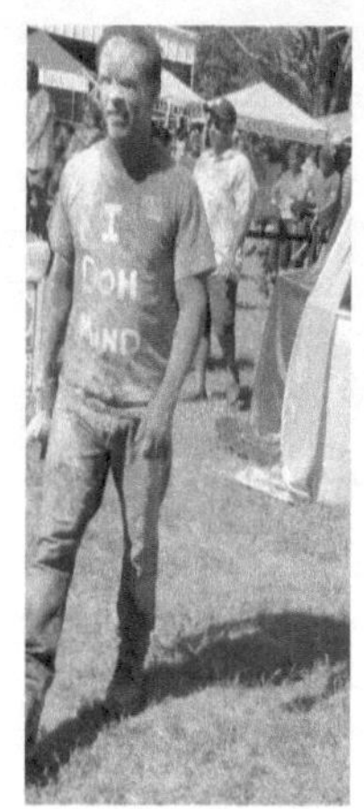

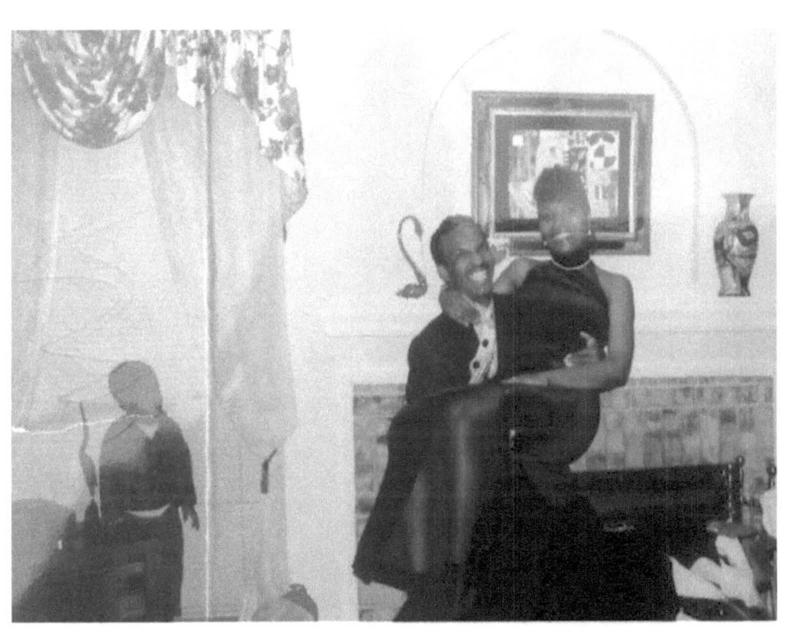

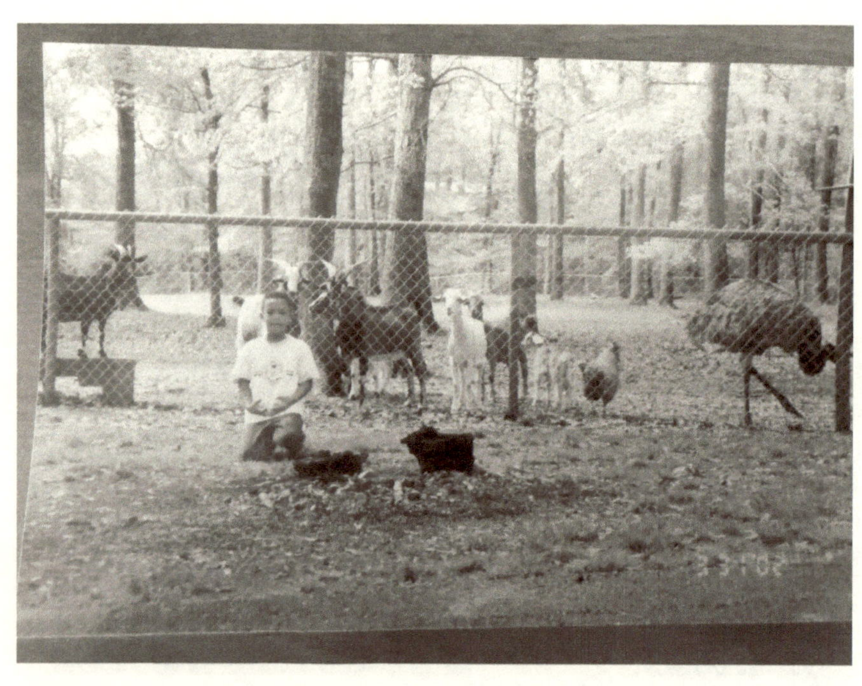

My Son Sterling at home with his element.

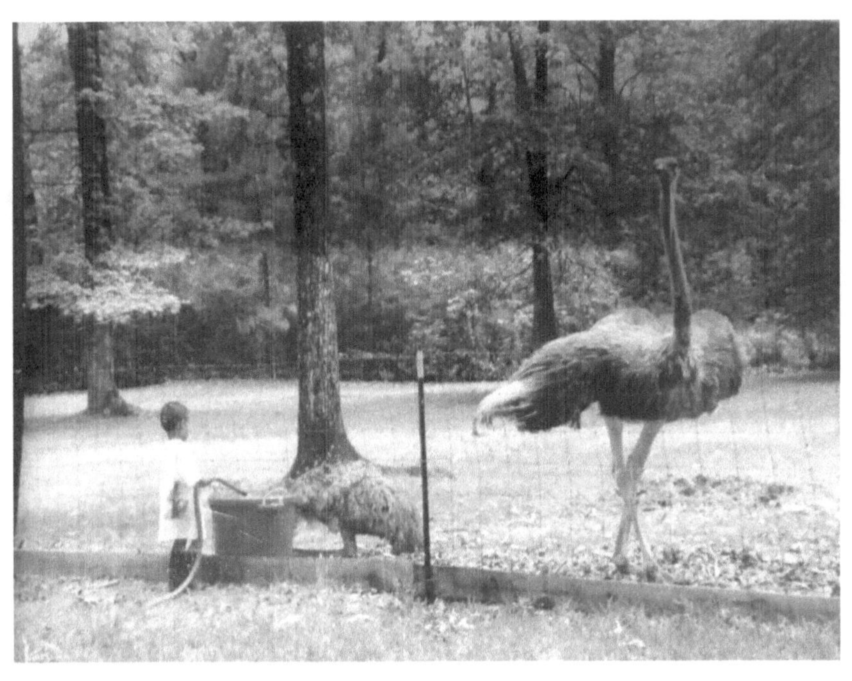

My Son at work!!!

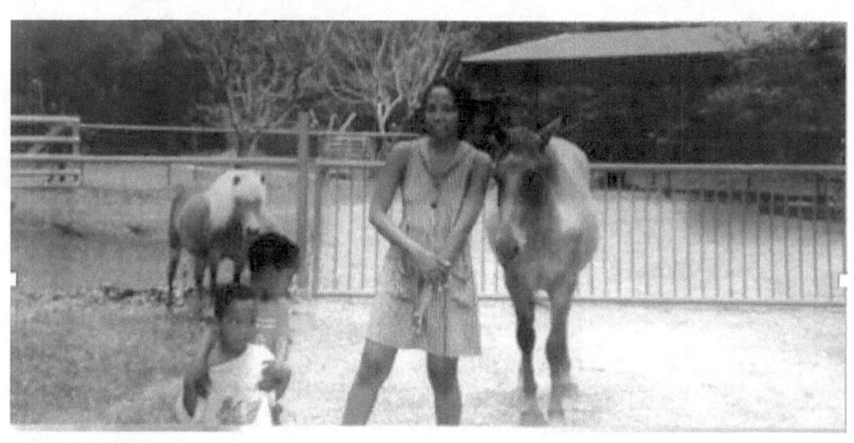

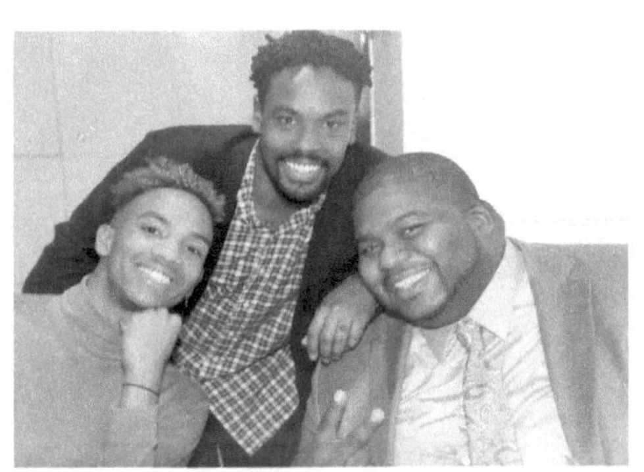

My 3 son's

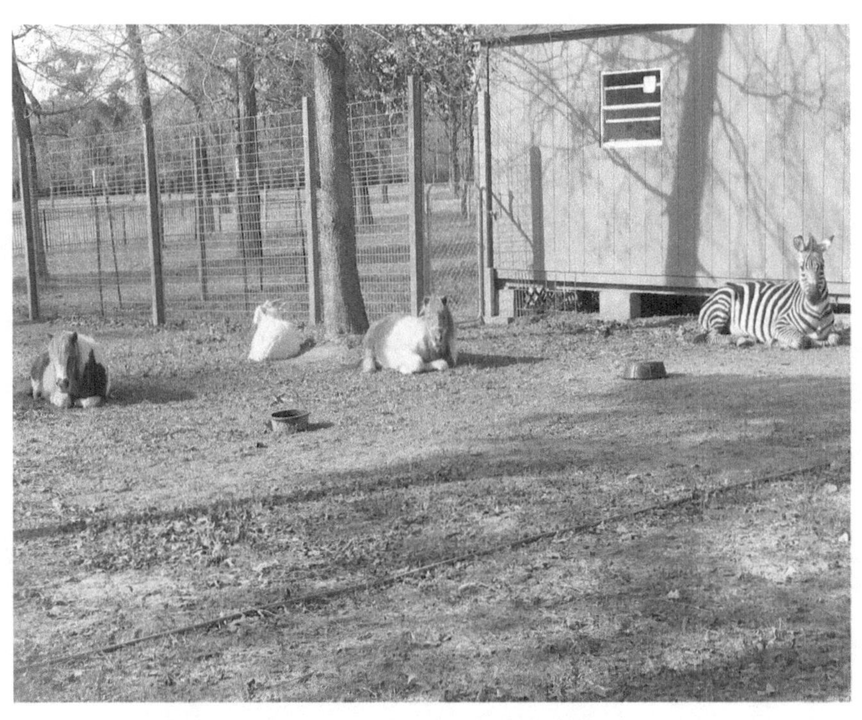

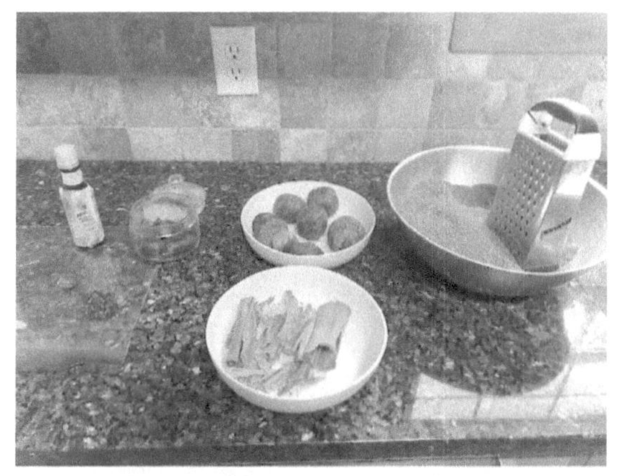

100% coca

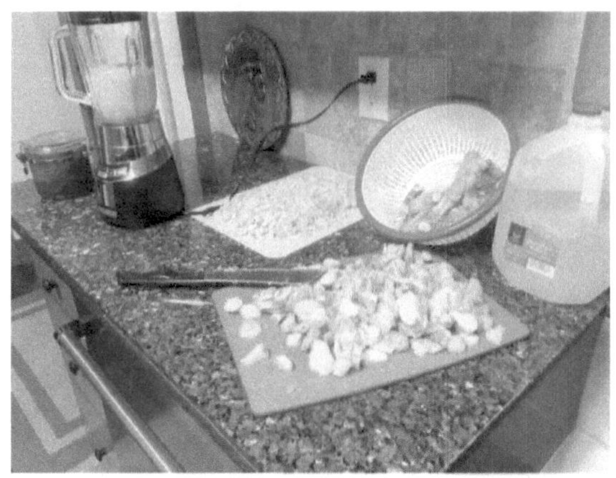

Preparing for Ginger Beer

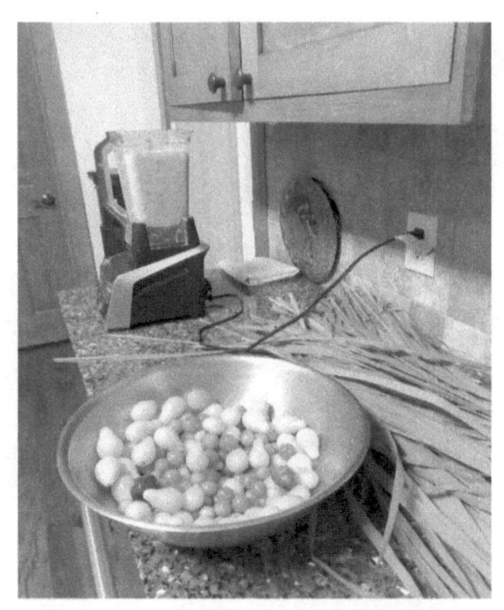

Fresh tomatoes sauce; lemon grass

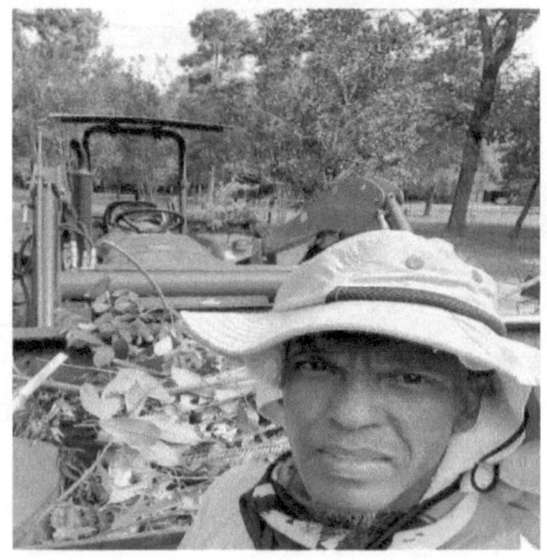

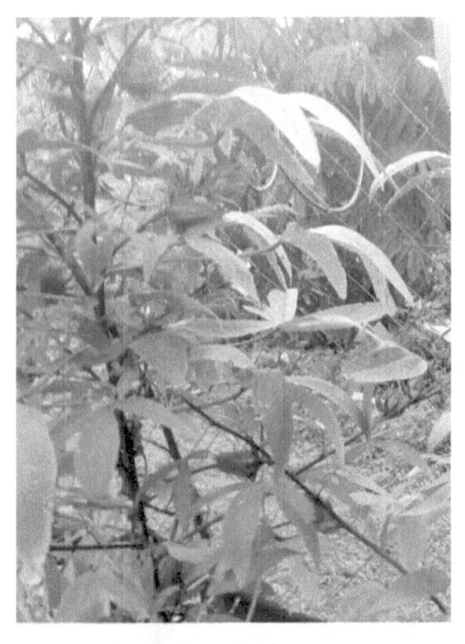

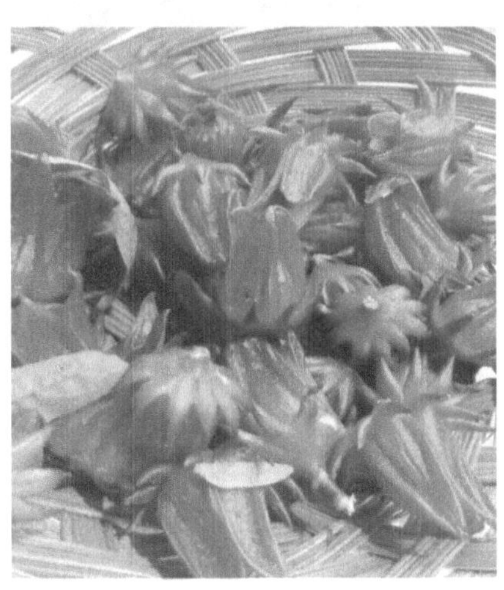

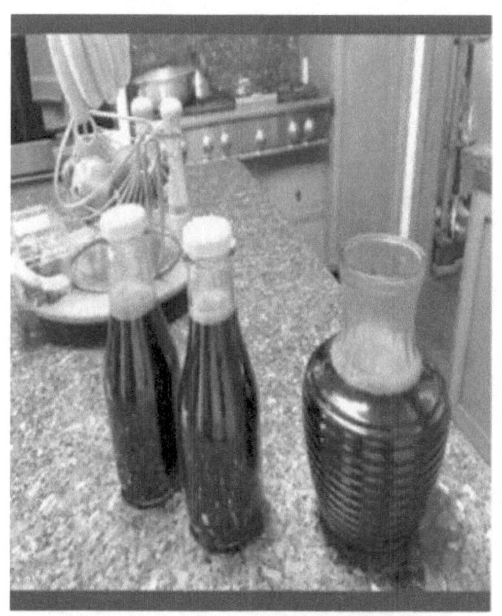

Hibiscus Roselle: Plant, Flowers & Juice (sorrel)

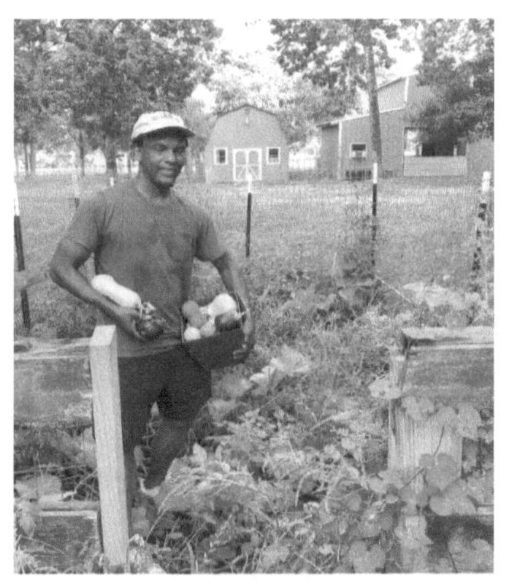

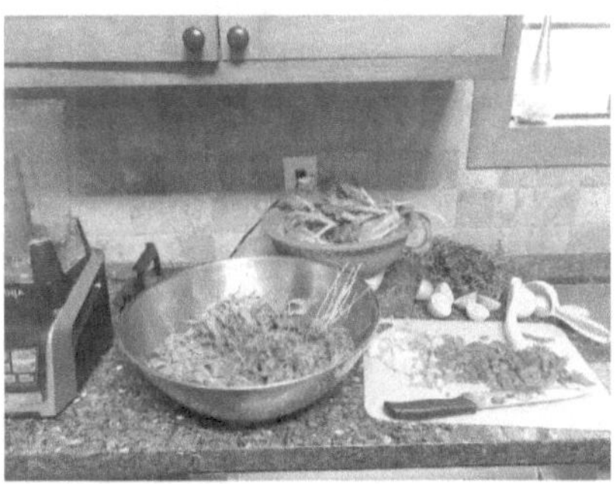

Variety of vegetables and herbs

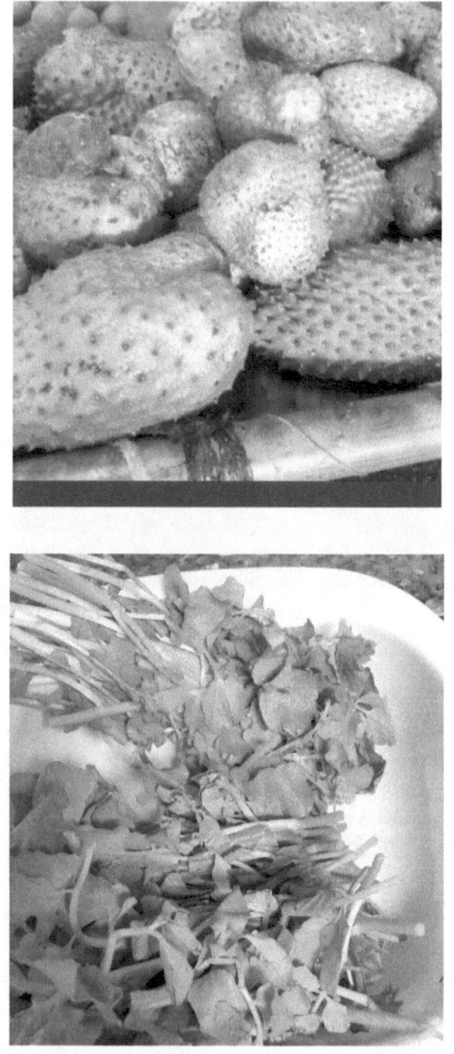

Super Foods: soursop and water cress

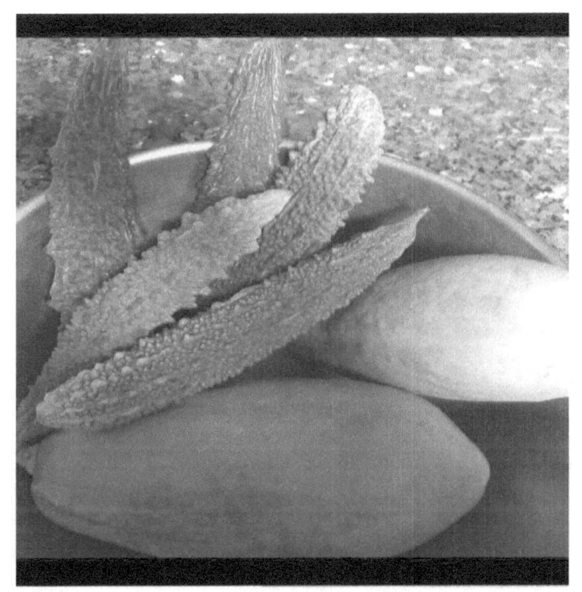

Super Foods: papaya and bitter melon

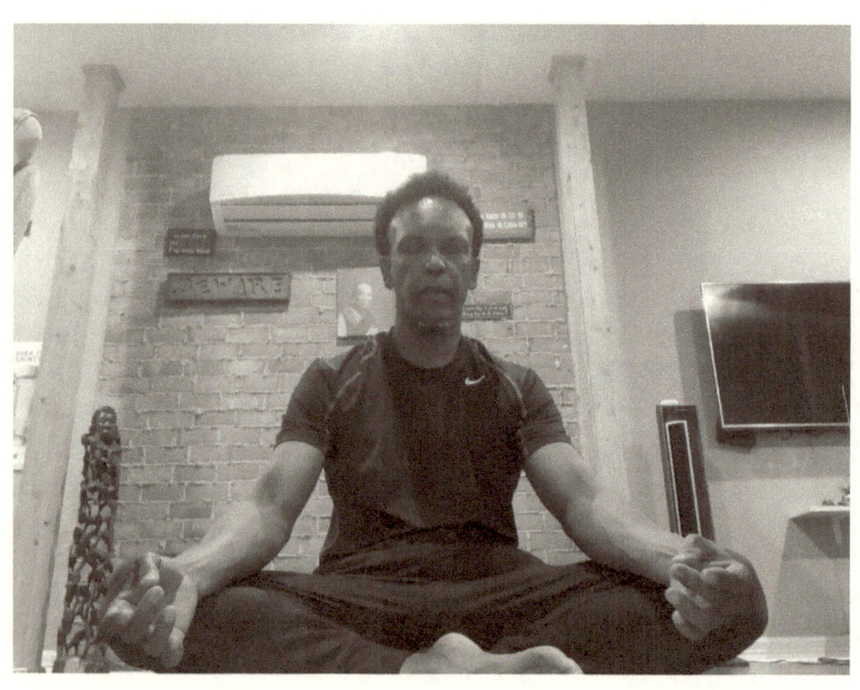

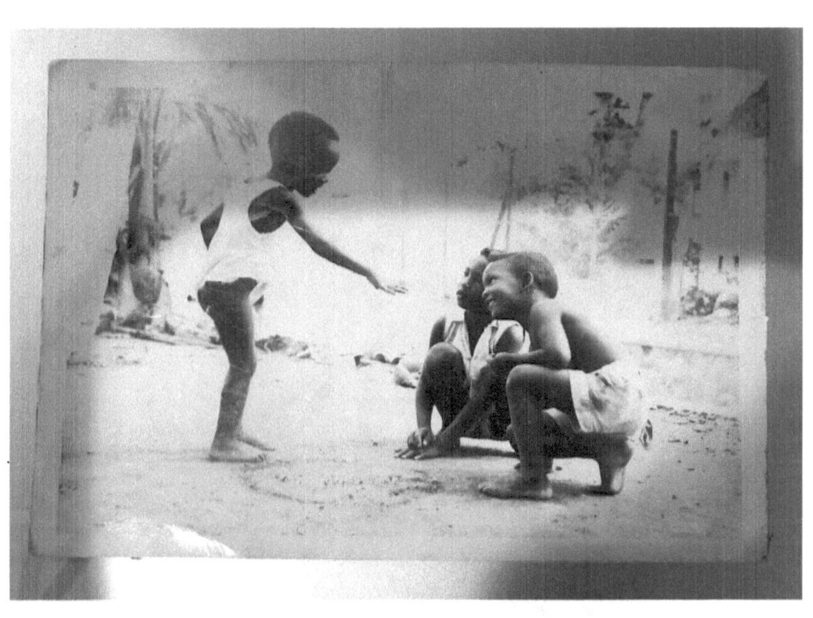

Left to right – best friend, my brother and I

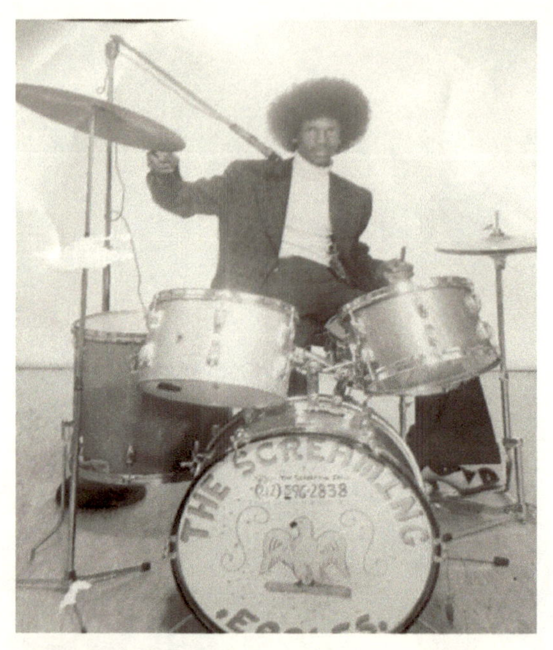
THE SCREAMING
(612) 596-2838
EAGLES

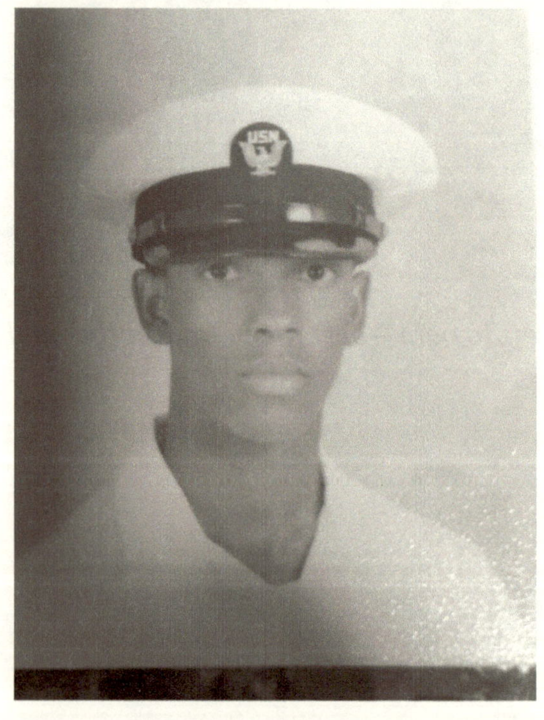
USN

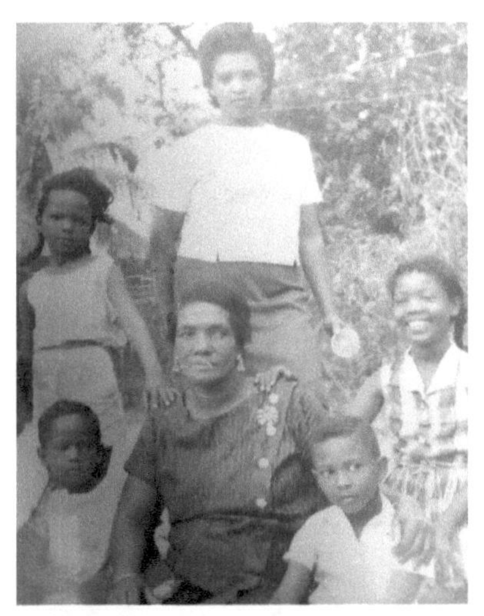

Top Center-clockwise:
Mother, sister, brother
grandmother,
myself and sister

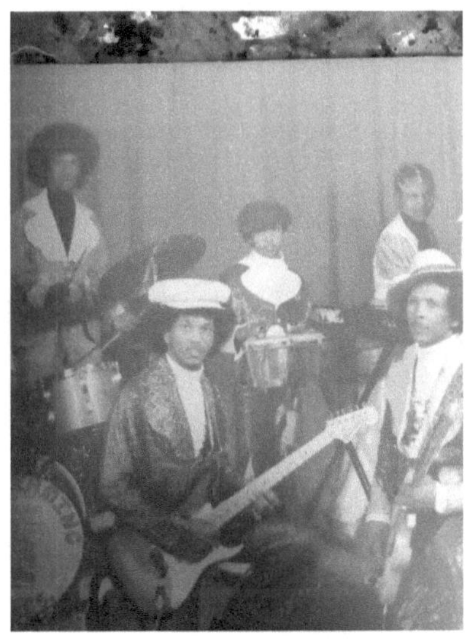

Family Band

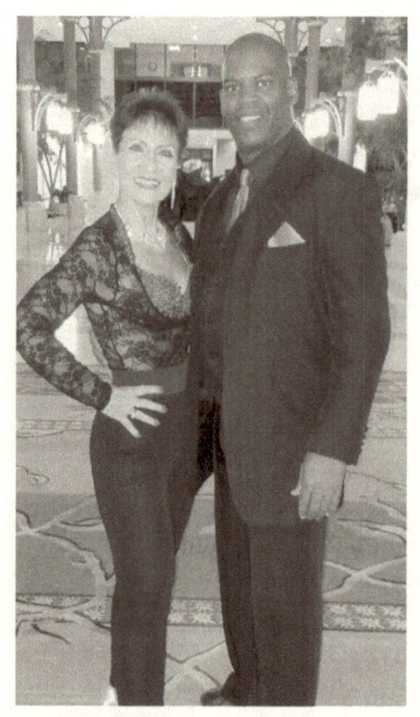

Raye Avery & Irene Griffin dance instructors (R&I Dance Studio)

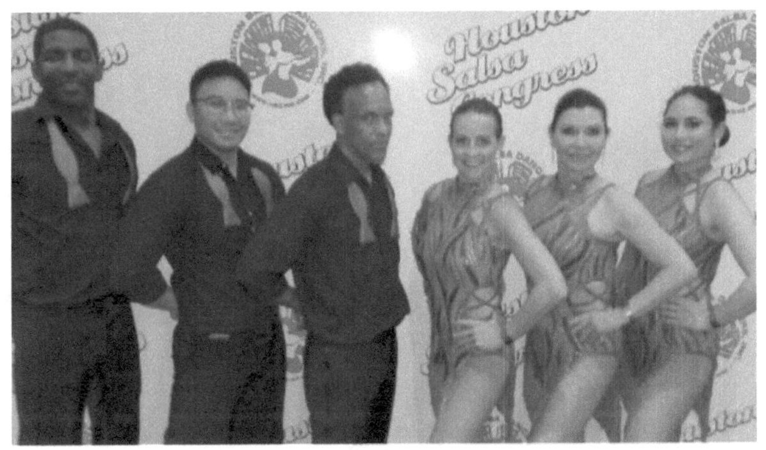

R&I Salsa Team 2020

*L-to-R: Quentin, Neal,
Myself, Christine,
Lauren and Stephanie*

BIBLIOGRAPHY

Bellwether Media. *Seeing: The Five Senses.* 1st ed. Minneapolis, MN: Bellwether Inc., 2018.

Claybourne, J. *The Usborne Complete Book of the Human Being.* United Kingdom: Usborne Pub Ltd., 2002. www.usborne-quicklinks.com.

Hever, J., and J. R. Cronise. *Plant-Based Nutrition.* 2nd ed. Indianapolis, IN: DK Publishing, 2018.

Jenkins, M. *Food Fight: GMOs and the Future of the American Diet.* New York: Penguin Random House, 2017.

Kurlansky, M., and S. D. Schindler. *The Story of Salt.* New York: G.P. Putnam's Sons, 2006.

McCathy, E., and M. Mulligan-Ewing. *Wine.* 7th ed. Hoboken, NJ: John Wiley & Sons, 2019.

Mindell, L. E., and V. Hopkin. *Prescription Alternatives: Hundreds of Safe, Natural, Prescription-Free Remedies to Restore and Maintain Your Health.* 4th ed. New York: McGraw-Hill, 2009.

Morrison, A. *Homegrown Honey Bees: An Absolute Beginner's Guide to Beekeeping; Your First Year, from Hiving to Honey Harvest.* North Adams, MA: Story Pub, 2013.

Randall, K. D. *Dreamland: Adventures in the Strange Science of Sleep*. New York: W. W. Norton & Company, 2012.

Sadhguru, J. V. *Inner Engineering: A Yogi's Guide to Joy.* New York: Spiegel & Grau, 2016.

Scharffenberger, J., and R. Steinberg. *The Science of Chocolate*. New York: Harry N. Abrams, 2005.

Sedgewick, A. *Coffeeland: One Man's Dark Empire and the Making of Our Favorite Drug*. New York: Penguin Press, 2002.

Weil, A. *Natural Health, Natural Medicine: The Complete Guide to Wellness and Self-Care for Optimum Health.* Rev. ed. Boston: Houghton Mifflin Company, 2004.

ABOUT THE AUTHOR

Tony Noreiga grew up in the Caribbean island of Trinidad and Tobago. Having migrated at the age of twelve, he has spent most of his life in the United States. Prior to college, he served four years in the United States Navy. He later graduated from Iowa Podiatric Medical School and has practiced as a foot surgeon for twenty plus years.

Life, Nutrition, and Wellness 101: A Holistic Approach with a Philosophical Twist is Dr. Noreiga's second publishing. His first book, published in 2018, is entitled *Fruit for Thought*.

www.ingramcontent.com/pod-product-compliance
Lightning Source LLC
Chambersburg PA
CBHW051451250726

48655CB00001B/348